SO-BXA-019

THE CARIBBEAN STATE,

HEALTH CARE AND WOMEN

THE CARIBBEAN STATE, HEALTH CARE AND WOMEN

AN ANALYSIS OF BARBADOS AND GRENADA DURING THE 1979 – 1983 PERIOD

PATRICIA RODNEY

RA 564.85
R63
1998

Africa World Press, Inc.

P.O. Box 1892

Trenton, NJ 08607

P.O. Box 48

Asmara, ERITREA

Africa World Press, Inc.

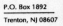

P.O. Box 1892
Trenton, NJ 08607

P.O. Box 48
Asmara, ERITREA

Copyright © 1998 Patricia Rodney

First Printing 1998
All rights reserved. No part of this publication may be reproduced, stored in a retrieval system or transmitted in any form or by any means electronic, mechanical, photocopying, recording or otherwise without the prior written permission of the publisher.

Cover and Book design: Jonathan Gullery

Library of Congress Cataloging-in-Publication Data

Rodney, Patricia.
    The Caribbean state, health care, and women : an analysis of
Barbados and Grenada during the 1979–1983 period / Patricia Rodney.
       p.   cm.
    Includes bibliographical references and index.
    ISBN 0-86543-516-2 (cloth). -- ISBN 0-86543-517-0 (pbk. : alk.
paper)
      1. Women's health services--Government policy--Grenada.
2. Women's health services--Government policy--Barbados. 3. Medical
policy--Grenada. 4. Medical policy--Barbados. 5. Women--Health and
hygiene--Grenada. 6. Women--Health and hygiene--Barbados.
    I. Title.
RA564.85.R63   1996
362.1'98'0972981--dc21   96-47412
                                                   CIP

DEDICATION

Dedicated to my three children:
Shaka, Kanini and Asha
and in loving memory of
my mother, Louisa Henry
my mother-in-law, Pauline Rodney
my dear friend and mentor Dame Nita Barrow.

CONTENTS

PREFACE xi
ACKNOWLEDGEMENTS xiii
INTRODUCTION xv

SECTION 1: LITERATURE REVIEW 1

CHAPTER 1: THE STATE IN CAPITALIST SOCIETIES
    FEMINIST PERSPECTIVES ON THE CAPITALIST STATE 3

CHAPTER 2: THE STATE IN THE PERIPHERY 21
    INDEPENDENT AND
    NATIONAL LIBERATION MOVEMENTS IN THE PERIPHERY:
    THE CONTEXT OF THEIR EMERGENCE 33
    THE POST-COLONIAL STATE IN THE CARIBBEAN 35

CHAPTER 3: WOMEN AND THE CARIBBEAN STATE 53

**SECTION 2: THE CARIBBEAN STATE,
HEALTH CARE AND WOMEN** 75

CHAPTER 4: EMPIRICAL RESEARCH METHODOLOGY 77
    SELECTION OF RESEARCH AREAS 77
    RESEARCH PROCEDURE 80
    METHODOLOGY & METHODOLOGICAL ISSUES 81
    RESEARCH CHALLENGES 85

CHAPTER 5: HISTORICAL OVERVIEW OF
    WOMEN'S HEALTH IN THE CARIBBEAN 89
    PRE-SLAVERY (1492-1643) 90
    SLAVERY (1644-1833) 91
    APPRENTICESHIP (1834-1838) 94
    FULL EMANCIPATION (1838-1900) 96
    PRE-INDEPENDENCE (1900-1960) 97
    POST-COLONIALISM/INDEPENDENCE (1960-1980) 103

CHAPTER 6: BARBADOS 109
    THE POLITICAL SITUATION 109

THE ECONOMIC SITUATION 114
THE STATE AND WOMEN 119
THE HEALTH CARE SYSTEM 125
    Health Infrastructure 125
    Health Care Financing 128
    Health Policy and Administration 130
    SUMMARY 138

CHAPTER 7: GRENADA 145
THE POLITICAL SITUATION 145
THE ECONOMIC SITUATION 154
THE STATE AND WOMEN 158
THE HEALTH CARE SYSTEM 163
    Health Infrastructure 163
    Health Care Financing 166
    Health Policy and Administration 169
    SUMMARY 176

CHAPTER 8: ASSESSMENT OF STATE HEALTH CARE
IN BARBADOS AND GRENADA:
THE PROFESSIONAL'S PERSPECTIVE 183
    GENDER SENSITIVITY 184
    BARRIERS TO HEALTH CARE SERVICES 189
        Middle Class Women 190
        Ability to Pay for Services 191
        Attitude of Service Providers 192
        Doctor-Nurse Relationships 194
        State Hospital Nurse-Polyclinic Nurse Relationship 195
        Consumer Involvement 196
        SUMMARY 199

CHAPTER 9: ASSESSMENT OF STATE HEALTH CARE
SYSTEMS IN BARBADOS AND GRENADA:
THE WOMEN'S PERSPECTIVE 203
    CONDITIONS OF EXISTENCE 204
    CRITIQUE OF THE HEALTH CARE SYSTEM 213
        1. Service Availability 214
        2. Service Satisfaction 217
        3. Service Accessibility 222
        4. Service Comparability to Private Health Services 224
        SUMMARY 229

SECTION 3: BEYOND THE STUDY 235

CHAPTER 10: CONCLUSION AND RECOMMENDATIONS 237
 THEORIES ON THE STATE: A SUMMARY 237
 BARBADOS AND GRENADA IN THE POST STUDY PERIOD:
 POLICY CHANGES AND REVERSALS 240
 FUTURE DIRECTIONS: RECOMMENDATIONS 240

BIBLIOGRAPHY 245

TABLE OF APPENDICES

Appendix 1: Map of the Caribbean 259
Appendix 2: Health System Components/Elements 260
Appendix 3: Detailed Demographic Profile of the
Barbadian and Grenadian Women Interviewed 261

INDEX 263

LIST OF TABLES

4.1 Barbados and Grenada: Selected Demographic
and Health Statistics 1979-1983 and 1984-1993 79
5.1 Life Expectancy at Birth (yrs) by Country, Region and Sex
1965-1975 and 1975-1980 105
6.1 Rate of Unemployment, 1982: Selected Caribbean Countries 117
6.2 Breakdown of the Health Budget in Barbados, 1979-1983
to the nearest million (Barabdos Dollars) 129
6.3 Manpower (Barbados): Health Personnel
with Population Ratio 1979-1983 139
7.1 Grenada Government Revenue and Expenditure,
1981 (US Millions) 156
7.2 Health Facilities in Grenada and its Sister Islands 167
7.3 Grenada, Selected Health Economic Indicators 169
7.4a Manpower (Grenada):
Health Personnel with Population Ratio, 1981 177
7.4b Manpower Distribution (Grenada):
Health Personnel Per Health District, 1981 178
9.1 Barbados and Grenada: Percentage Distribution of Population
Fifteen Years and Over by Educational Attainment
(Highest Level Attended) and Sex, 1980-1982 208
9.2 Critique of State Health Care by Barbadian and Grenadian
Working Class Women: Comparative Summary Of Findings,
1979-1983 and Post 1983 231

LIST OF FIGURES

6.1 Map of Barbados: Location of Polyclinics
and other Health Facilities 127
7.1 Map of Grenada: Location of Health Centers
and other Health Facilities 165

PREFACE

This book developed from a study designed to examine the levels of efficiency and adequacy of state health care policy and service provision with respect to women during the 1979 to 1983 period in Barbados and Grenada, two small post-colonial states in the English-speaking Caribbean. These two countries were selected because of:

1. The different socio-political development paths (and health policies) pursued by these two States during the 1979 to 1983 period;
2. The uniqueness of Grenada's revolution experiment; and
3. The lessons to be learnt from the two types of health care models implemented, including the different strategies used in the development of primary health care programs and service delivery.

Primary Health Care (PHC) as advocated by the 1978 Alma Ata Declaration is "the first level of contact with individuals, the family and community with the national health system, bringing health care as close as possible to where people live and work, and constitutes the first element of a continuing health care process."[1]

The main purposes of this project were to determine the role of the State in the provision of health care services to working class women and the impact of these services on the health of the women. Secondarily, it examined whether in either State, women participated in all/or some aspects of health care policy development.

The results of the data analysis utilizing primary and secondary sources revealed that the health care services provided to working-class women in both Barbados and Grenada during the period 1979 to 1983 was neither "holistic" nor "gender sensitive," but rather was based on a medical "ill-health" model and focused primarily on women's reproductive health. Although both countries instituted Primary Health Care (PHC), albeit by different routes and with different outcomes, Grenada seems to have come closer to realizing the model of health care advocated by the Alma Ata Declaration of 1978. Grenada appeared to have focused (more than Barbados) on health education and promotion efforts through the active involvement and participation of the consumers, the aim being to democratize the health system and demystify medicine. However, although these efforts were commendable and could be considered "progressive," women in general worked longer hours and were given more responsibilities. They also lacked the related power necessary to institute serious change.

Based on its findings, the study recommends the development of services for the Caribbean that are more "women-centered" and "reality" based, encompassing all aspects (influencers) of health (as defined by the WHO). One concept of consumer oriented/sensitive and issue/needs based planning can be found in the District Health Council model operative in Ontario, Canada.

The District Health Councils are local coordinating and planning bodies made up of interdisciplinary representatives including consumers. Use of a participatory model by Caribbean States would promote internally developed services and programs that focus on the "holistic" health needs of women.

Notes

1. Report of the International Conference on Primary Health Care, Alma Ata, Russia "Alma-Ata, Primary Health Care." Geneva: WHO, 1978:3-4.

ACKNOWLEDGEMENTS

The completion of this project would have been more difficult without the love and support of many people. I especially want to acknowedge Shaka, Kanini, Asha, Delly and Al.

I am indebted to the Barbadian and Grenadian women who willingly shared their time, experiences and gave me permission to use their "voices." I appreciate the assistance extended to me by the health care providers and professionals in both States. To the staff of the libraries and resources centers in Barbados and Grenada: Caribbean Council of Churches, Central Bank of Barbados, Caribbean Development Bank, Pan American Health Organization (PAHO), UNICEF, ISER, UWI Cave Hill, WAND and Marryshow House who assisted me in locating important documents.

Special thanks to my thesis committee: Professors Nora Ceboratev, Budd Hall, Gordon West (supervisor); George Dei (chair); Rudy Grant (external examiner); and Hilary Beckles (field advisor).

Extreme gratitude is due to my original editoral team Kanini Rodney and Cedric Licorish, and to Pat Winfield for administrative support, Abeo Jones, Natalie Kanem and Phyllis-Jones Changa for assistance with the final corrections and editing.

I was fortunate to receive the assistance of Elias Amare Gebrezgheir, Staff Editor at The Red Sea Press, and Kassahun Checole, Publisher of Africa World Press and The Red Sea Press, who believed in the project.

Last but not least, the International Development Research Council (IDRC) Canada whose financial assistance made it easier to do the research.

P.R.
Atlanta, GA.

INTRODUCTION

FOCUS OF THE STUDY

This study sought to examine state health policy and its impact on women's health, specifically that of working-class women within two Caribbean[1] states with significantly different socio-political development paths: Barbados under the BLP, and Grenada under the PRG. The period of study selected was from 1979 to 1983.

The decision to study Barbados and Grenada during the 1979 to 1983 period was based on a number of reasons. Most significant was the change in political ideology that Grenada underwent during the Revolutionary (1979 to 1983) period and the effects this had on the development of socio-economic and health policies during that time. This transition was compared to the much smoother one of Barbados. Grenada State refers to mainland Grenada as well as its sister islands, Carriacou and Petit Martinique. Both states, recognizing the need to better serve their respective populations, and in response to other internal and external influences, adopted Primary Health Care (PHC) in accordance with the Alma Ata Declaration in 1978.[2] The participants at the 1978 International Conference on Primary Health defined primary health care as "essential care based on practical, scientifically sound and socially acceptable methods and technology made universally accessible to individuals and families in the community through their full participation... It forms an integral part both of the country's health care system, of which it is the central function and main focus, and of the overall social and economic development of the community. It is the first level of contact of individuals, the family, and the community with the national health system, bringing health care as close as possible to where people live and work, and constitutes the first element of a continuing health care process."[3] This study, in its assessment and comparison of Barbados and Grenada, illustrates how two post-colonial states, with different approaches to their socio-economic, political, ideological and cultural development, assumed different aspects of PHC and promoted superficially different (though fundamentally similar) health care models.

Policy development in the Caribbean, as in most other developing and developed countries, has been subject to gender, race, class and social inequities. Traditionally, policies have been designed by men with little regard for, or understanding of, women's concerns and the consequences of these policies on women's health and well-being. The study highlights this point, showing in both cases how inappropriately health policies dealt with women's issues; in fact, the state was instrumental in making women "invisible." By investigating the development and subsequent implementation and management of health policies by the two states and focusing directly on the women's views about the state's policies, the study attempts to understand existing inequities. Included is an assessment of women's participation in the political and administrative processes and in the development and implementation of policies that affect their well-being. In addition, the resulting health status of women is examined in the context of the socio-economic and political situation of each state. In effect, the study evaluates the strengths and weaknesses of each state with regard to their ability to adequately service women's needs.

There is a general tendency for women's health to be confined specifically to issues related to motherhood and reproductive health (the reproductive organs, menstruation and childbearing). Although these issues are important, they do not encompass women's entire reality. "Women have both general health needs, the same as the rest of the population, and health needs that are specific to them as women."[4] For the purpose of this study, health is defined as "a state of complete physical, mental and social well-being and not merely the absence of disease and infirmity."[5] In addition several factors, including race, age, social and economic status, ideology, geographic or regional location, the physical environment, politics and health policies,[6] are now known to contribute to the overall health of an individual and should be considered in the development of an adequate health care system. Accordingly, the study has explored each state's defined health philosophy and examined fiscal and policy frameworks that supported their philosophy as well as the extent to which health policies were incorporated into the broader socio-economic development policies: political will of government in implementing their policies; support of the medical establishment; and political consciousness of the civil society in making sure that these policies are enacted.

These analyses were amplified by a critique of the system by a group of professional men and women. These findings were used to examine the differences in policy development in each state and assess inequities inherent in the system. The developments that occurred in the health sector during the 1979 to1983 period were situated in perceptions of Barbadian and Grenadian working class women who were interviewed about the system's ability to meet their needs. Working class women in the sample also gave their views of the policy changes, contrasts and reversals that occurred after the study period (collapse of the revolution and death of Maurice Bishop, and the U.S. intervention in Grenada in 1983; and after the death of Tom Adams in 1985 and the subsequent defeat of the BLP in Barbados, in 1986).

SIGNIFICANCE OF THE STUDY

This socio-historical analysis of health care systems in two English-speaking Caribbean countries revealed a number of similarities generated from similar colonial and post-colonial experiences.[7] In the colonial period, the focus of the health care system was on curative services provided through predominantly urban-based hospitals. People in rural areas were treated at "dispensaries" (similar to outpatient clinics) which operated on a weekly or monthly basis and were designed to treat mainly the indigent. Public health measures were mostly confined to containing and treating epidemic and endemic diseases such as malaria, tuberculosis, hookworm and other communicable diseases.

During the colonial period, the development of policy was usually done extra-regionally and had very little input from nationals who actually worked within the system. As such, the public policy failed to address the primary health care needs of the vast majority of the Caribbean working class people. Sir Frank Stockdale, the first Comptroller for Development and Welfare in the West Indies, may be viewed as visionary since he challenged the system, in his 1940-42 report, "to promote the health of the whole population while continuing to adequately care for the sick."[8] Prior to independence, there was still no coherent policy for the development of health care services in the region. Each government appeared to tackle the problem of basic human needs by responding to crises in different sectors of the economy, whether they involved the lack of health or housing facilities or employment. The adjustments made to the health care systems were based, not only on the country's socio-economic situation, but on the priority each state placed on health and health care, and the political will of those with power. Despite the state's historical attitude to health and health care, the policy structures built were heavily influenced and conditioned by the relationship with the dominant metropolitan power given the continued socio-economic and political dependent status of the colonies.

After independence, major improvements were made in the health sector. These were attributed, in part, to the following strong but complementary forces: political pressures put on the governments by Caribbean peoples; important lobbyist roles played by individual 'local' public health specialists throughout the region; and subsequent changes made in public health policy. Gains were made in areas such as maternal and child health (specifically in immunization and nutrition) which, combined with positive changes in socio-economic conditions, contributed to a reduction in the infant mortality rates and an increase in life expectancy at birth within the region.

However, although definite strides were made in health (some at the primary health care level), there remains a definite focus on curative measures remained. There was a lack of formal and informal health education and promotion programs which emphasize preventive measures that are gender specific. Consequently, women continue to suffer high morbidity rates from preventable diseases such as hypertension, anemia and obesity.[9] As will be shown, women's health has been jeopardized by diverse influences such as legal rights, education, employment, housing, social class, occupation, food and nutrition and environmental factors. Some of the underlying causes of women's health problems and factors that influence the extent and the nature of morbidity are malnutrition, poverty, homelessness, fatigue, overwork, stress, violence and exploitation;[10] yet, women's health care programs continue to ignore these factors and continue to be tied mainly to their reproductive/productive roles.[11]

Interestingly enough, although many health problems plaguing women are preventable and although these facts are well known by the health experts and political and economic powers within the region, eradication of the root causes has not been adequately addressed and solutions have not been conveyed to the public at large. In effect, these institutions seek to maintain their control and protect their interests and these concerns take priority over resolving women's health issues.

This study specifically addressed two states in the Caribbean and refrains from drawing broad conclusions about other Caribbean countries or developing nations even though there may be some common themes. It is an innovative project in that it investigates, analyzes and compares state health policy in Barbados and Grenada (before and during the 1979 to 1983 period) and is supported by both qualitative and quantitative data from primary and secondary sources which highlight the impact of these policies on women and their health. The research leads to the formulation of a number of suggestions and future policy directions to address women's health needs, and to improve their overall health status. It is contended that such an undertaking would require structural changes in the societies in question. These changes would require long term political commitment backed by public persistence to keep the issues alive. As an original study, it provides a basis for further discussion, research and development. Hopefully, it will contribute to policy change in the Caribbean as pertains to women in all aspects of their lives.

OBJECTIVES OF THE STUDY

1. Determine the role of the state in the provision of health care in Barbados and Grenada highlighting the changes that occurred in the health care system during the period 1979 to 1983;
2. Ascertain whether, in either State, women participated in some or all aspects of the development of health care policy and state policy in general;
3. Assess the perspectives and views of government and non-government personnel about health services and reform in Barbados and Grenada from 1979 to1983;
4. Identify the specific health care needs of Barbadian and Grenadian women, particularly those of the working class (as articulated by these women themselves), and determine the effectiveness of the health care services in addressing these needs;
5. Identify some of the advances and/or reversals in (health policy) that took place in Barbados and Grenada at the end of the period under investigation;
6. Produce a set of recommendations and suggestions for future policy directions that would inform policy makers, planners and women's organizations.

To achieve the above objectives, two strategies were used: (1) a theoretical framework was developed to analyze the Caribbean State, specifically Barbados and Grenada, and how the State functioned and developed policies, particularly vis-à-vis women; and (2) a multidimensional methodology was used to examine the health care system of these two Caribbean states.

ORGANIZATION OF THE STUDY

The study consists of three sections organized as follows:

Section 1: LITERATURE REVIEW

Chapter 1: The State in Capitalist Societies: a review of the pertinent literature on the typologies of State formation in capitalist societies, including a feminist perspective.

Chapter 2: The State in the Periphery: a comparable review of the literature on the State in the periphery, with an emphasis on Caribbean societies.

Chapter 3: The State and Women in the Caribbean: provides a theoretical overview of the literature on women in the Caribbean.

Section 2: THE CARIBBEAN STATE, HEALTH CARE AND WOMEN

Chapter 4: Empirical Research Methodology: details the methodology used in the study.

Chapter 5: Historical Overview of Women's Health in the Caribbean: provides a historical overview of the socio-economic and health conditions of Caribbean women from slavery to the post-colonial and independence periods and a look at the development of State health care policy and systems.

Chapter 6: Barbados: provides an overview and analysis of the State's political, socio-economic and health care systems during the period 1979 to 1983.

Chapter 7: Grenada: provides an overview and analysis of the State's political, socio-economic and health care systems during the period 1979 to 1983.

Chapter 8: Assessment of State Health Care Systems in Barbados and Grenada: The Professional Perspective: a critique of health policy and health care systems in Barbados and Grenada using the professional perspectives of administrators, planners and providers.

Chapter 9: Assessment of State Health Care Systems in Barbados and Grenada: The Women's Perspective: gives detailed background information about the Barbadian and Grenadian women interviewed, followed by their critical analysis of the health care systems.

Section 3: BEYOND THE STUDY

Chapter 10: Conclusion and Recommendations: Summarizes the theories of the State and its influence on policy; specifically health policy as it relates to working class women. Briefly looks at the health care system in the two States during the period 1984 to 1993; draws conclusions about the State's ability to meet the health care needs of working class women; and recommends preliminary steps towards improving the health status of Barbadian and Grenadian women, particularly those of the working class.

Notes

1. Sometimes still referred to as the West Indies.
2. "Alma Ata Primary Health Care" Report of the International Conference on Primary Health Care, Alma-Ata, Capital of the Kazakh Soviet Socialist Republic, USSR: jointly sponsored by the World Health Organization, (WHO) and UNICEF, Geneva: 1978; see also Convergence, International Journal of Adult Education, Toronto, Canada, Vol XV, No. 2, 1982:14.
3. Alma Ata 1978:16.
4. Patricia Smyke. *Women and Health*, London and New Jersey: Zed Books Ltd. 1991:3.
5. World Health Organization definition, see Clair Blackburn *Poverty and Health: Working with Families* : Milton Keyes, Philadelphia: Open University Press, 1991:31.
6. See Hilary Graham (1984); Doyal, Lesley (1983); Patricia Smyke (1991) and Agnes Miles (1991).
7. See Eric Williams (1970); RS. Sheridan (1985).
8. Sinha, Dinesh P. *Children of The Caribbean 1945-1984: Progress in Child Survival, Its Determinants and Implications,* Jamaica: Caribbean Food and Nutrition Institute (PAHO/WHO), 1988:125.
9. see E R. M. Le Franc (1990).
10. Agnes Miles (1991); Rhoda Reddock (1989), Hilary Graham (1984).
11. See Jane Cottingham (1984); WHO Report, (1985):5.

SECTION 1:
LITERATURE REVIEW

This section reviews some of the available literature on the State and women in order to gain an understanding of the interrelationship between the two and, more importantly, to get a sense of how women are perceived by the state. The primary concern of this section is the State and women in the English speaking Caribbean; however, given that the Caribbean is enmeshed within the international and capitalist system, some of the more general theoretical formulations on the State are pertinent to this discussion.

The review begins with a look at pertinent literature on the State in capitalist society, including a feminist perspective which not only critiques some of the gender-based and patriarchal assumptions but also suggests alternative ways in which women's relationship to the state should be viewed. Chapter 1 feeds directly into the next in that it highlights the underlying assumptions on which the post-colonial peripheral state is based and, consequently, has been analyzed. Chapter 2, thus, examines the literature on the state in the periphery, with emphasis on the Caribbean. Chapter 3, which builds on the framework provided in Chapter 2, focuses more specifically on work done on the State and Caribbean women.

The literature review presented, though not exhaustive, provides a basis from which one can begin to (1) examine the development of State health policy and health care systems in the English-speaking Caribbean; (2) assess the impact of these policies and structures and systems on the health of Caribbean women; and (3) examine more recent health policy and service delivery developments in the Caribbean, and particularly in Barbados and Grenada.

However, in order to accomplish the aforementioned tasks, a more complete appreciation of the State is necessary. This can only be achieved through a systemic examination of the historical context of the State in the Caribbean, paying attention to how the political and socio-economic systems are developed. This will be done in Section 2.

CHAPTER 1

THE STATE IN CAPITALIST SOCIETIES
FEMINIST PERSPECTIVES ON THE CAPITALIST STATE

Discussions on the capitalist state, which were neglected in the early post-war era (an era dominated by American intellectual hegemony), have re-entered the arena over the past two decades "giving rise to a proliferation of theoretical and empirical analyses on specific aspects of the state apparatus and state power."[1] Major contributions to the debate on the state were the works of Ralph Miliband and Nicos Poulantzas produced in the 1970s, these culminated in a theoretical and historical debate. "The "Miliband-Poulantzas debate" played a key role in stimulating the interest in the anglophone world but many other currents, American as well as European, fed into the same theoretical stream."[2] It is important to note that (notwithstanding the insistence of Third World scholars for historical specificity when studying the periphery) the structural connection of the periphery to international capitalism suggests that the debate itself would be incomplete without consideration of the relationship between the capitalist and peripheral states and an understanding of how the state functions and is defined. In discussing the State, a number of questions immediately come to mind—the answers and interpretations of which will enhance the reader's perspective and interpretation of the State. For example, one may need to determine if the state is best defined in terms of its legal form, its repressive and ideological apparatus, its institutional composition and boundaries, its mode of operation, its declared aims and its forms and functions for the broader society or alternatively, one may examine its sovereign place in the system of international capitalist relations or still one may ask if a combination of both aspects form the best approach to conceptualizing the State. Further, one may query whether "the state is a thing, a subject, a social relation, or simply a construct which helps to orientate political action."[3] According to Jessop,

> the core of the state apparatus comprises a distinct ensemble of institutions and organizations whose socially accepted function is to define and enforce collectively binding decisions on the members of a society in the name of their common interest or general will.[4]

At another level, some writers who seek to develop explanations of the state in terms of its form, functions, content and role in society, despite dissimilarities and variations in their positions, seem to agree that the state assumes a very important role in mediating and regulating not only class conflict, but also many areas of political, socio-economic and cultural life. This latter point was explicitly formulated from a British stance in the following passage below which, though lengthy, underscores this central emphasis:

> You may turn on the radio for the news; an agency accountable to Parliament may (depending on the station) provide it, interpret it, affect the way you see the world. You may see the children off to school: whether or not it is a state school, what they are taught there is regulated by the state, at least to some extent....If you travel by public transport, the state

provides it or regulates it....suppose your place of
work is an industry or firm: whether or not the state
actually owns it, the state exerts a great variety of
powerful influences on it—as regulator, licenser, sub-
sidiser, standard setter, rate-setter, taxer, buyer, seller-
and thereby affects your life at work. The state
influences the level of images, the value of money, and
the cost of credit you need to buy a television set in
order to watch programs conforming to government
regulations in the evening.... [Therefore]....it [is] hard
to think of more than a few aspects of daily life that
are not affected by decisions and regulations of the
state....[Apart from] the provision of services and their
regulatory aspects for the entire community....state
agencies also choose. They make decisions that can
benefit some people, and hurt others....state agencies choose when they use force to control certain
individuals and groups [and not others] in the name of
"maintaining law and order."[5]

The significant point to note here is that, in terms of class and
gender, the groups that dominate the process of regulation,
mediation, choice and provision are overwhelmingly ruling class
and male. Given the historical processes of domination and subordination that have characterized the conditions of women's
lives, the parameters within which women's struggles and relations have been articulated need to be stretched.

MacKinnon in discussing the "political" in her formulation on
the state refers to it as an autonomous entity that is affected and
constrained by the economic structure of society though not
reducible to it. For her, the state, is "relatively autonomous";
that is, the state is expressed through its functionaries, has a definite class character, is definitely capitalist or socialist, but also it
has its own interests, which are to some degree independent of
those of the ruling classes and even of the class structure."[6]

O'Connor, in his conceptualization of the capitalist state,
contends that it is the

undemocratic and bureaucratically organized "executive branch." The formally democratic "representative branch" is defined as the "government." Elected

representatives who constitute the government formally make the laws.... The bureaucratic organisation of society's working bodies...means that neither individual citizens nor their representatives are responsible for carrying out public work themselves. Citizens are institutionally and legally prevented from learning to regulate their own social affairs democratically.[7]

He further shows how in the United States,

the state is pluralistically organised, i.e., it consists of semi-independent and independent bureaucracies which are "relatively autonomous" not only in relation to capital but also in relation to one another. This state pluralism and associated system of "interest group liberalism" have been the main vehicles for political competition between capitalist enterprises and factions and the class struggle between capital and labour.[8]

Apart from the pluralist position, the Marxist theory of the state in the Poulantzas-Miliband debate, stimulated considerable analysis and interpretation of the capitalist state and its concomitant relations. Ollman, for instance, working within a Marxist analytical framework, has advanced eighteen theses to explain the capitalist state and its related dynamics. Among them is the notion that

it is conceived of as a complex social relation of many different aspects, the main ones being political processes and institutions, the ruling class and an objective structure of political/economic functions, and an arena for class struggle.[9]

While Ollman tried to describe the capitalist state in terms of a set of complex social relations, Miliband saw the state in more instrumental terms. In a rather simplistic Marxist view, he regarded the state as an instrument of the capitalist class. Another Marxist, Poulantzas, attempted a more sophisticated structural analysis of the state in capitalist society, positing that it is an arena of class struggle and class contradictions.[10]

Other Marxist scholars in dealing with the problematic of the state have advanced analyses based on assumptions derived from Gramsci's, and designed to "break with the cruder forms of state theory and develop more sophisticated analyses of the capitalist state and its role in social reproduction."[11] What seems to appeal to many of them are the arguments Gramsci advances against economism, suggesting that one cannot reduce questions of political practice to those concerned with the mode of production or fundamental economic relations.[12] Gramsci was concerned to show that

> the state was a class force which had a vital role in the organization of class domination, in securing the long-term interests of the bourgeoisie, as well as its unification, in facilitating concessions to the subordinate classes and in securing the active consent of the govern (in parliamentary democracies) or effecting their demobilization (in more despotic forms of the State). This means that the working class must build its own organs of political power and state power.[13]

Gramsci's view of *hegemony* becomes very important for understanding the workings of the capitalist state. The concept of hegemony was elaborated on to include the practices of a capitalist class or its representatives, both in gaining state power and in maintaining that power once it has been achieved. Gramsci distinguished between domination and intellectual and moral leadership:

> A social group can, indeed must, (already exercise "leadership" before winning governmental power); it subsequently must continue to 'lead' as well.[14]

The concept of hegemony has been transformed by Gramsci from a strategy into a practical tool for understanding society in order to change it. Hegemony is a relation between classes and other social forces within society; a hegemonic class or part of a class is one which gains the consent of other classes and social forces through creating and maintaining a system of alliances by means of political and ideological struggle.[15]

Many scholars, therefore, have sought to utilize the premises of these Marxist points of departure for their analyses and studies. Thus these theoretical insights also have enhanced our understanding of the characteristics and dynamics of the capitalist state. Despite these useful contributions, it is difficult to agree on a definition of the state for two main reasons. First, as pointed out by Jessop, any existing state comprises a multiplicity of multifunctional institutions and organizations

> which have at best a partial, provisional and unstable political identity and operational unity and which involve a complex overdetermined dynamic. Thus differences can legitimately arise as to which particular features are treated as primary or definitive and which secondary or contingent.[16]

Secondly,

> discounting the complexities of states themselves, differences also arise because the concept of the state has a central role in political life itself. This holds not only for disputes about the boundaries, purposes and limits of any given state but also for processes of state-building and reorganization intended to transform that state. This suggests that the concept is not just essentially contested but also that dominant conceptions can influence the nature of the state itself. [17]

This difficulty and reluctance that Jessop has in formulating a clear definition of the state is evident when he states that:

> States are not the sort of abstract, formal objects which readily lend themselves to a clear-cut unambiguous definition, nor are they suited as the starting point of a general theory of politics or socialization. Thus it is not a proper job for state theorists to offer a definition which specifies once and for all the abstract, formal characteristics of the state. Instead it is their task gradually to build up an understanding of the state as a form-determined social relation through a steady spiral movement from abstract to concrete and from simple to complex. Inevitably this movement can never be completed: it would always be possible to make any account more concrete and more

complex. And, as this progressive movement towards an analysis of the state which is ever richer in theoretical determination proceeds, previous assumptions, principles and concepts will be continually redefined.[18]

Feeling somewhat compelled to move beyond the observations above concerning the difficulties involved in formulating a definition of the state, Jessop for his own clarity attempts to develop a plausible comprehensive definition in the following manner:

> ....any general definition of the state would need to refer to state discourse as well as state institutions.... The core of the state apparatus comprises a distinct ensemble of institutions and organizations whose socially accepted function is to define and enforce collectively binding decisions on the members of a society in the name of their common interest or general will. This broad 'cluster' definition identifies the state in terms of its generic features as a specific form of macro-political organization with a specific type of political orientation; it also establishes clear links between the state and the political sphere and, indeed, the wider society."[19]

Thus Jessop contends that:

> rather than provide a spuriously definitive general theory of the state apparatus and state power in capitalist societies what is important is to construct a theoretically-informed and realistic account of specific phenomena that result from a complex synthesis of multiple determinations.[20]

Finally, while Jessop's perspective has been strongly influenced by Marxist assumptions, he has seen the importance of reformulating a number of these in order to avoid "all forms of reductionism." In effect, Jessop does not attempt to reject "fundamental Marxist insights into the character of the state as a system of political class domination ... [Instead the perspective] does require a careful specification of the conditions in which insights hold true."[21]

Connell's critique of "mainstream State theory" differs. Connell argues that classical theories of the state are unhelpful in the sense that they have failed to adequately and directly address the issue of gender:

> The liberal tradition that discusses citizenship, property, personal rights and the rule of law presents the "citizen" as an unsexed individual abstracted from social context.[22]

Connell, further contends that the socialist, anarchist and Marxists perspectives on the state are also problematic when dealing with questions concerning gender:

> socialist and anarchist analyses of the state as an agent of domination add in social context, but only in the form of class; the contending classes seem to be of all the same sex. [23]

Concerning the neo-Marxists discourse on the state, Connell asserts that the class emphasis which forms the main part of this perspective does not address adequately issues of gender.

> the concept of the relative autonomy of the state is concerned with autonomy from class interests only, the radicalism of Marxist state theory is severely comprised by its gender blindness....The analysis of the state as an agency of class power is based on a specific conception of "class"; this rises from a political economy which excludes domestic production, therefore much of women's work, for calculation. [24]

Connell referred to the "patriarchal state" as a system of domination by men over women, noting that:

> the term is much debated; it has been criticized in particular for a false universality, attributing modern Western patterns of men's domination over women to the rest of the world and the rest of history. This implication can and should be dropped. In that case, "patriarchy" is a serviceable term for historically-pro-

duced situations in gender relations where men's domination is institutionalized; embedded in face-to-face
settings like the family and the workplace, generated
by the functioning of the economy, reproduced over
time by normal operation of schools, media and
churches. Prejudice is part of this, but only a small part
of the whole. [25]

Another concern of Connell was "how we should study men in
gender relations and what view of modern world history an
understanding of masculinity might give us."[26] Contemporary
changes in masculinity should be seen "not as the softening (or
hardening) of a unitary "sex role," but as a field of institutional
and interpersonal changes through which a multilateral struggle
for hegemony in gender relations, and advantage in other structures, is pursued."[27]

He further notes that,

The distinctive feature of the present moment in gender relations in first-world countries is the fact of open
challenges to men's power, in the form of feminism
and to institutionalized heterosexuality, in the form of
lesbian and gay men's movement. We must distin-
guish between the presence of these movements from
the operating power they have won, which is often
disappointedly small. Whatever the limits to their gains
and the success of the conservative backlash, the historic fact these movements are here on the scene
structures the whole politics of gender and sexuality
in new ways.[28]

Feminist Perspectives on the Capitalist State

Feminists have also been attempting to examine state structures
both in advanced capitalism and in the dominated and dependent
periphery. The bulk of this literature has been recently produced
and its importance lies in the fact that it strives to grapple with
issues pertaining to women's lives that previously have been
either inadequately treated or ignored. In referring to "feminists,"
it is important to note that we are not a homogeneous group,

and that we in fact belonging to different social classes and political/ideological orientations.[29] This point is important when dealing with the realities of black people's struggles, particularly with regard to those which have significant relevance to this study and the Caribbean women it addresses.

At a general level most feminists argue that the state, as it is constituted presently, does not adequately represent women's concerns.[30] MacKinnon in her examination of the analyses offered by Marxist and liberal feminist writers stated that

> feminism has a theory of power but lacks a specific theory of its state form, Marxism has a theory of value which through the organisation of work in production becomes class analysis, but also a problematic theory of the state. Marx himself did not address the state much more explicitly than he addressed women. Women were substratum, the state epiphenomenon.... Engels frontally analyzed women and the state, and together. But just as he presumed the subordination of women in every attempt to reveal its roots, he presupposed something like the state, or state-like society, in every attempt to find its origin.[31]

A number of radical Marxist feminists have argued that Marxism constituted an important theoretical and methodological perspective that focused on the relations of exploitation and appropriation. However, as argued by Barrett, the systems of concepts that it employs "do not and could not directly address the gender of the exploiters and those whose labour is appropriated."[32] Barrett further states that Marxism's analysis of capitalism was "conceived around a primary contradiction between labour and capital and operated on a 'sex-blind' level."[33]

MacKinnon recognized that there were flaws and weaknesses in both the liberal and left theories and concluded that feminism was left with only two alternatives. Either (1) the state is viewed as a primary tool of women's betterment and status transformation, without analysis (hence strategy) of it as male; or (2) women are left to civil society which, for them in any case, has more closely resembled a state of nature.[34]

Feminists further contend that the state in capitalist society has a different impact on women than on men.[35] Armstrong &

Armstrong provide a vivid description of the pervasiveness of the state in women's public and private lives.

> Women are employed by the state; they are clients of the state; they appeal to the state for protection and redress. The dominant ideology and women's ideas about themselves are influenced by the ideas perpetuated in state institutions, by organizations of state structures and services, by the structure of state policies and practices. [36]

Burstyn, and other feminists, have attempted to examine "the state and the ways in which it acts as an organizer and enforcer of male supremacy"[37] and to demonstrate

> the importance of the state in maintaining and enforcing women's financial dependence on men and in supporting and legitimating the various dimensions of women's oppression in .... society.[38]

They concluded that:

> the state plays an important role in contributing to the oppression of women, especially those women in the periphery who are most exploited and oppressed by, and subordinated to, the relations of peripheral capitalism that have been dominated by men through its own specific structure and operation.[39]

The above arguments presented by feminists reflect views of the metropolis. However, these same points are relevant to an understanding of Caribbean societies as well, notwithstanding the specific historical differences of these societies relative to those of the metropolis.

According to a number of women working within a feminist framework, the existing literature on the state has tended to devote insufficient or inadequate attention to the relationship between gender and other forms of exploitation, dependency, and structural inequality produced and reproduced on the basis of such factors as class, race, ethnicity and religion within the Third World states.[40] A number of reasons are posited for this neglect or absence of serious account of women's struggles, experiences, class functions and positions within these societies.

Fatton noted that in Africa the

> ....ruling classes exist throughout....but that they have yet to become hegemonic. Their domination and their rule express more the threat and use of direct violence than their moral, material, and intellectual leadership. Ruling classes are in the process of constructing their hegemony; in their quest they are using gender as a means to consolidate the classes. While still fluid and in flux, entry into the ruling class is increasingly difficult and virtually blocked to independent and autonomous women.[41]

Fatton further argues that within African states

> the construction of ruling class hegemony has the effect of conflating male power with class closure. Women are not totally excluded from the ranks of ruling class, but their quest for status and wealth depends inordinately on aligning themselves with powerful men. In the absence of such alignments women tend to withdraw from the public arena to build their own parallel and independent spheres of survival. The emancipation of women is thus linked to the struggle against ruling class hegemony; it requires both a feminist and a class consciousness.[42]

This view is supported by Elabor-Idemudia whose study of rural Nigerian women revealed that "factors of women's incomes, household expenditure and marketing, nutrition, health care and decision-making show a general deterioration in women's access to and/or control over the factors." [43] She further stated that:

> In the Nigerian political scene, women are not only under-represented but their issues and concerns are not taken seriously....Where women do occupy positions of political leadership, they are members of the ruling class and subservient to their husbands who placed them there.[44]

Secondly, even within the progressive movements, women's concerns are often ignored or overlooked because of the "pressing needs and direction of the struggle."[45] Although many men may verbally express identification with women's concerns, in reality they have difficulty questioning the very assumptions with which they exercise power in political parties, social movements, and other organizations and institutions.[46]

Thirdly, Claire Robertson contends that even though some women have obtained a certain level of independence from male dominance, this position is difficult to maintain in changing economic circumstances.

> ....[W]hile many women aspire to the male dominated elite, most will remain in female networks where they are economically independent from men, and poor as a consequence....That women have been able to survive so far has largely depended on the strength of those networks. However, socio-economic forces are weakening that strength and making it logical for younger women to trade off economic independence for the anticipatory greater security of dependence on man.[47]

Fourthly, there are many women who, by virtue of their subordinate position within the class structure, have become marginalized. That is they are:

> ....segregated or excluded in varying degrees, from full participation in society. They are denied equal access to opportunities which the state makes generally available, and in some cases are effectively excluded from such participation in social and political life as is commensurate with the normative standards of society....needless to say, the extent and form of state intervention in delimiting opportunity and access, and in legislating to deny former "rights," varies according to the social standing and political power of such groups.[48]

The argument advanced by feminist writers (some of whom have strongly identified and integrated themselves into the struggles and forms of resistance of the masses of women in the Third World) has recognized the importance of analyzing women's struggles with rigorous theoretical tools. However, MacKinnon identified a key deficiency in the feminist discourse on women and the state. She concluded that "feminism has no theory of the state," and supports this with the following three points: [49]

1. Feminism has not confronted, on its own terms, the relation between the state and society within a theory of social determination specific to sex. As a result it lacks an explicit jurisprudence, that is, a theory of the substance of law, its relation to society, and the relationship between the two. Such a theory would comprehend how law works as a form of state power in a social context in which power is gendered.
2. Feminist practice has oscillated between a liberal theory of the state on the one hand and a left theory on the other. Both theories treat law as the mind of society: disembodied reason in liberal theory, reflection of material interest in left theory.
3. Liberalism applied to women has supported state intervention on behalf of women as abstract persons with abstract rights, without scrutinizing the content and limitations of these notions in terms of gender.

Feminism, in its attempt to counter the economic reductionist discourse which failed to address the fundamental realities of gender exploitation and domination,

> points in a different direction, emphasizing precisely the relations of gender—largely speaking of the oppression of women by men—that Marxism has tended to pass over in silence.[50]

Thus, to the extent that Marxists focused on the state and its ideological and repressive apparatuses, feminists argued for emphasis to be placed "on the specific character of gender relations."[51] To achieve this, one must have a framework that is

> capable of exploring the relations between the organization of sexuality, domestic production, the household, their material and social conditions of life and so on; and the historical changes in mode and relations of production and systems of appropriation, exploitation and subordination.[52]

Armstrong and Armstrong have attempted to show that, because the debate has moved "beyond the question of the relationship between household and formal economy to involve a range of issues, including sexuality, resistance and power,"[53] both Marxist analyses and the categories of political economy need to be approached critically if they are to be meaningful, and thus, contribute to an understanding of women's position in advanced capitalist society. They further contend that some writers have advanced the position that the fundamental assumptions of political economy

> preclude an analysis of women, and some have held that two distinct explanatory frameworks—one for "reproduction" and one for production—are necessary, others have maintained that the political economy approach has to be stretched, not by adding women to it or by focusing exclusively on women, but by making the theory in general more sex-conscious. [54]

However, Dahlekrup argued that this is only possible if the state is carefully analyzed,

> The state is not one unified block....[so] if political actors.... like the women's movement, or questions of intentions and motives are involved, a more specific understanding of the state is necessary. We must look upon local, regional as well as national politics and we must look at conflicting interests within the state.[55]

The state is not autonomous or mechanistic in form but it represents the collective expressions of the "dominant and dominated classes." Women also are not a homogeneous group but represent both dominated and dominant groups although it could be argued that women's lack of state power prevents them from realizing gender equality and independence.

The above analyses of the capitalist state by liberal, Marxist and feminist scholars revealed that the state is predominantly patriarchial and gender-blind. The end result is the lack of representation of women's concerns which reinforces women's dependence. This unfavorable effect is due to the fact that the state impacts differently on women than on men.

These findings, although useful, need to be further examined to ascertain (a) whether the experiences of women in the periphery are similar and (b) some of the additional problems experienced by women in post-colonial states.

Notes

1. Jessop. State Theory:U.K. Polity Press, Cambridge Journal of Economics, 1990:338.
2. Ibid. For more details on the Miliband-Poulantzas debate read Miliband, R. *The State in Capitalist Society*. New Left Review:1968).
3. Ibid.:349.
4. Jessop:1990:341.
5. *Politics, Legitimacy and the State,* Open University Press, London:1982,Units 14 &15:9-10.
6. Catherine A. MacKinnon. *Toward a Feminist Theory of the State*: Harvard University Press, 1989 :158.
7. James O'Connor. *The Fiscal Crisis of the State:* New York St. Martin's Press, 1973.
8. Ibid.
9. Bertell Ollman. "Theses on the Capitalist State." *Monthly Review* :1982,34: 7:40.
10. See Poulantzas. (1969); See also Miliband (1970); Ollman (1982).
11. Bob Jessop(1990) :142.
12. Ibid.:145.
13. Ibid.:106-107.
14. Roger Simon. Gramsci's Political Thought. London: Lawrence & Wishart, 1992:22-24.
15. see Ibid.:22-23.
16. Bob Jessop, UK.(1990):339.
17. Ibid.:339-40.
18. Ibid.:341.
19. Ibid.:341.
20. Bob Jessop. *The Capitalist State:Marxist Theories and Methods* New York:University Press, 1981:259.
21. Ibid.:259.
22. R.W. (Bob) Connell. "The State in Sexual Politics: Theory and Appraisal.":Mimeo, 1989:2.
23. Ibid.
24. Ibid.:3.
25. Ibid.:6.
26. Ibid.:2.
27. Ibid.
28. Ibid.:14.
29. See J Mitchell and A Oakley. *What is Feminism*: Oxford,

Blackwell, 1986; Roxanna Ng, "Introduction" *Women, Class, Family and the State.* Varda Burstyn and Dorothy E. Smith. Toronto:Garamond Press, 1985 and others.
30. see Burstyn and Smith 1985; Armstrong and Armstrong (1991) and others.
31. Catherine A. MacKinnon. *Towards a Feminist Theory of the State*: Harvard University Press, 1987:.17.
32. Michele Barrett. *Women's Oppression Today.* London:Verso Books,1988:8.
33. Ibid.
34. Catherine A. MacKinnon (1989):160.
35. Hugh Armstrong and Pat Armstrong. *Theorizing Women's Work.* Toronto:Garamond Press,1991.Melanie Randall. *"Feminism and the State: Questions for Theory and Practices."* *Resources for Feminist Research*:1988:10-16; Varda Burstyn, Dorothy Smith(1985); Dorothy E. Smith. *Feminism and Marxism* Vancouver:New Star Books,1977.
36. Hugh Armstrong and Pat Armstrong.(1991):113.
37. Varda Burstyn and Dorothy Smith.(1985):45
38. Ibid.
39. Ibid.:227.
40. See Kathleen A. Staudt and Jane L. Parpart(1990);see also Linda Carty and Dionne Brand(1988);Bell Hooks(1984); Maxine Molyneux(1987);Angela Davis(1980).
41. Robert Fatton. "Gender, Class and State in Africa." *Women and the State in Africa* (eds.) Kathleen A. Staudt and Jane L. Parpart:1990,p.48.
42. Ibid.:48.
43. Elabor-Idemudia, Patience."Rural women's Quality of Life Under Structural Adjustment Policy and Programmes: A Nigerian Case Study." Unpublished Ph.D. dissertation,1993:209.
44. Ibid.
45. Andaiye,"Women in Political Parties." *Caribbean Contact*.Barbados:August,1988 .
46. See Andaiye(1990); see also Maranda Davies. *Third World's Second Sex.* London and New Jersey: Books Ltd 1983, Vol.22nd.ed.
47. Kathleen A. Staudt and Jane L. Parpart (1990)
48. Tom Chapman and Juliet Cook. "Marginality, Youth and Government Policy in the 1980s." Critical Social Policy, 22:Summer 1988:44.
49. Catherine A. MacKinnon(1989):157-160.
50. Michele Barrett(1988):8.
51. Ibid.:9.
52. Ibid.

53. Hugh Armstrong, and Pat Armstrong. *The Practical Guide to Canadian Political Economy.*Toronto: James Lorimer Company, 1985.
54. Ibid.
55. Drude Dahlekrup. "Confusing concepts - Confusing reality: a Theoretical Discussion of the Patriarchal State." Anne A. Sasson, (ed.) *Women and the State.* London: Hutchison, 1987:110.

CHAPTER 2

THE STATE IN
THE PERIPHERY

While the literature on the state in capitalist society is extensive, the literature on the state elsewhere is relatively fragmented and underdeveloped. In the Caribbean particularly, the area to which this study is devoted, there are few rigorous analyses of the colonial and post-colonial state that use appropriate theoretical and methodological tools. The literature with respect to women and their relationship to the state in the Third World has not been fully developed to any significant degree, although there has been some progress made in recent times. The Caribbean still suffers from such deficiency and neglect. This fact is partly due to the inadequate treatment of women's issues and conditions of existence as a whole.

In the Third World, the state cannot be simply regarded as an impartial executor of some homogeneous national will, for these countries

> have been constructed, frequently by colonial rulers, from heterogeneous cultural traditions and social groups with divergent interests. In addition, states represent the interests of the different groups within a

nation unevenly. The state is, thus, rarely the un-contradictory proponent of a single group within society. The social nature of the state, in other words, is generally complex and contradictory.[1]

Crow further asserts that the nature of the state cannot be "read off" from the structure of an economy but there are significant differences between the interests of social groups associated with different forms of production, and differences in the way that those interests are expressed.[2]

Michel-Rolph Trouillot argues that, in most of the so-called Third World social formations, there is a tendency for the state to be unpredictable and unstable because of the "many inherent tensions to which it is constantly subjected."[3] Indeed the structural instability of the state is inherent in the social structure of peripheral capitalism, and it is produced from the dependent and subordinate characteristics of these societies themselves. Summarizing these features succinctly, Truillot writes:

> Societies on the periphery of the capitalist world economy are of necessity outward-looking, if only because they are economically dependent on capitalist centres. Yet states are inherently inward-looking (even if expansionist); they exercise primary control over a definite territory and derive their momentum from the dynamics of coercion within the space....the peripheral capitalist state is often a colonial legacy, the result of a political "independence" built upon the remains of a power structure imposed from outside.... The "national" state so created never inherited a blank slate because the preceding colonial entity, as well as the conditions of its demise, limited both new rulers' possibilities and those of their successors.[4]

Within the periphery of international capitalism and divisions of labour, the colonial and post-colonial formations have revealed a number of important features that have influenced H. Alavi into asserting that the "colonial mode of production" has resulted in a structural system of exploitation and domination that effectively undermines autonomous capitalist development. He identified these features as:[5]

- heavy concentration on *export* activities with emphasis given to raw material and semi-processed agricultural (as opposed to industrial) products;
- high expenditures on both *imported* necessities and luxury goods that are consumed by the numerically small but economically and politically dominant local bourgeoisie and required for production for export, e.g. oil;
- the retarded development of full capitalist relations of production in agriculture; comparatively low productivity of peasant and semi-proletarian labour (except in the case of Nicaragua);[6] and
- widespread backwardness in overall scientific and technological development.

Alavi argues that the colonial states exercised domination over all indigenous social classes and had their basis within the metropolitan centre itself. However, at independence the post-colonial societies inherited state apparatuses that were "overdeveloped" in relation to their class structures.[7] Having been freed from direct metropolitan dominance and control

> those at the top of the hierarchy of the military bureaucratic apparatus of the state are able to extend their dominant power in society, particularly with respect to the weak indigenous bourgeoisie. Therefore, the state has the autonomy to mediate the competing but no longer contradictory interests and demands of the propertied classes led by the metropolitan bourgeoisie.[8]

Simon, unlike Alavi, suggests that the post-colonial state is a relatively autonomous structure:

> at the same time that it mediates dominant class interests, the state acts on behalf of all propertied classes to preserve the social order in which their interests are embedded. That is, the state upholds the institutions of private property and promotes the capitalist mode as the dominant mode of production. The state also appropriates a large part of the economic surplus and invests it in bureaucratically directed economic activity. It thus assumes a relatively autonomous economic role....The strength and autonomy of the bureaucracy derives from this combination of administrative con-

trol and mediation, and the direction of many public agencies. [9]

He also provides another important perspective on the functions of the state in the post-colonial period by claiming that the state, and its various branches and organs serve to create favourable conditions for international and domestic capital accumulation

> not least through regulating the relations of production and social reproduction. The state also regulates the terms of external relations, although transnational corporations (TNC) exercise an often powerful influence. [10]

Simon adds that within the general literature on the post-colonial state in Africa, some writers assert that:

> African states are characteristically weak or "soft" in terms of institutional and policy implementation capacity and the often personalized nature of the government... (however) increased centralization and bureaucratic control have been the norm since independence. The extent of ossification, inefficiency and often also nepotism and corruption cannot be denied, whatever the legitimizing ideology, but it is crucial to appreciate that almost everywhere there has been at least a partial, if not total, coalescence of economic and political power in the hands of a small minority. In other words, state power has often been (ab)used by the new political elite to attain an often high degree of economic control, commonly in alliance with the growing indigenous economic elite...thus stifling weak and still commonly underdeveloped economies. Under such conditions, the politics of theft has also sometimes become rampant. [11]

Despite the internal contradictions that are produced in Third World societies which give rise to capital accumulation among some states, emerging groups are unable to develop into a strong bourgeoisie since massive amounts of capital are necessary to develop the productive forces of these societies. Further, because of the external structural barriers and restrictions that are imposed on these states with respect to capital, markets, technology, machinery, machine tools, agriculture implements, vehicles, and so on, the conditions for emergence of a powerful, autonomous capitalist class within the international division of labour are effectively blocked. The peripheral state, then, within advanced capitalism is fundamentally a weak state, and given the existing relations of production, is incapable of reproducing conditions to facilitate the development of the masses of people.

The fact, however, that a number of attempts have been made to explain the complexity of the state structures in the Third World does not necessarily mean that any distinct theoretical approach to the state has developed within these societies. Rather, Cypher argues that a theoretical perspective that draws from a number of salient and rich contributions to the discussions seems to be more appropriate than any one specific world-view dominating the analysis.[12] Thus he writes:

> The very dynamism and unpredictability of the economic system would seem to argue against any one theory of the state. Yet a case can be made for combining the instrumentalist theory (where the state is analyzed as an instrument of the ruling class), the relative-autonomy-of-the-state-theory, and the theory of state monopoly capitalism....These are complementary theoretical constructs that can be alternatively employed or emphasised in a given historical conjuncture. In other words, the state itself has no constant composition in terms of its degree of autonomy or instrumentality or in terms of the precise manner in which it intertwines with the accumulation process. As the latter is subjected to a greater or lesser degree of stress, as the process of socio-economic reproduction varies in terms of difficulty in time and place, the state is forced to respond. This occurs not in any mechanical and preordained manner but with structurally new combinations of the elements that can be derived from the three principal theories of the state. At any given point in time, one will most likely find elements from all three theories playing a role in defin-

ing the nature and parameters of the state construct.[13]

In fact Cypher seems to recognize that in his genuine attempts to avoid any reductionist or simplistic analysis of the state in the periphery, he is immediately confronted with a dilemma that suggests that the state structures in these societies are very complex. He therefore elaborates:

> It is no simple task to move adroitly among these three theories, plucking the most significant elements from them to present a model of the state....The question remains whether forming a conjunctural synthesis of the three dominant theories of the state is sufficient given that all have arisen from discussions of the nature of the state in purely capitalist modes of production. Whether one needs a particular theory of the state in conditions of what might loosely be defined as 'peripheral capitalism' remains an unfinished discussion.[14]

Cypher concludes that the answer to his theoretical dilemma lies in the rigorous, concrete historical analysis of the state in order to avoid any "crude approximation."

> [W]e are dealing with the relative weights of combinations, a fact that only becomes manifest when we turn to concrete historical situations.[15]

While the analysis advanced by Cypher poses some fundamental questions relating to the discussions on the state(s) in the periphery, Roxborough insists that

> ....any analyses of the state in the Third World must examine the mechanisms and institutions through which social classes have access to, and influence on, the making of state policy.[16]

In spite of the complexity of the state structures in the Third World, it is important to note

> that the dependent nature of these societies has revealed a number of similar tendencies when they are analyzed in the context of international capitalism.

These countries are economically dependent on the advanced capitalist world for loans, investment funds, technology, raw materials, capital equipment, spare parts, and in many instances, after independence, personnel to run the State apparatus. Thus, the imperialist powers can, by "cutting off the flow of these elements, cause not only severe economic damage but serious political problems as well."[17]

In the periphery where the state has a critical role, it may control the main source of revenue, and combine in its arrangement

the normal repressive state function with that of coordinator and organizer of economic life and the first-hand collector of the surplus. This makes the state, or rather those who are in control of it, relatively independent of traditional sources and supports of state power. The state and its controllers enjoy freedom to act, to suppress and to manoeuvre which would be unbearable in a normally productive society.[18]

Given the historical formation and development of the state in the periphery and its continued links to capitalism and imperialism, it remains in a subservient capacity which makes structural transformation of relations of domination and dependence extremely difficult. However, as Mansour notes, what is occurring in many Third World societies in the post-independence era is the consolidation of bureaucratic and dependent state capitalism.

It is state capitalism because the state.... [is] prime mover of all societal economic activity.... It is a special form of state capitalism since it is incapable of renewing, let alone extending, its productive base.... It is, of course, a dependent state capitalism. Nationalization notwithstanding, the producing and distributing transnationals still largely control the flow of surplus to the state and influence in important ways its economic and other decisions. Also, the state apparatus has been historically designed and shaped in such a way as to make of it essentially the link between local economic and social elements and the central imperialism, the tool for ensuring by all the means at the disposal of the state, including the repressive ones, that the former are subservient to the global interests of the latter.[19]

In the Third World under the dominance of colonialism there was no significant transition to self-sustaining capitalist development; no revolutionary transformation of the relations of production really took place, so in the post-colonial period "the state continues to function in the context of a plurality of dominant, propertied classes."[20] For example, in Pakistan:

> where a dependent or peripheral capitalist mode of production is grafted on to modified feudalism, three dominant classes have been identified, leaving aside their factions. These are the landlords, the indigenous bourgeoisie and the metropolitan bourgeoisie, none of which has managed to establish a controlling influence over the state apparatuses. The situation has made possible the emergence of a strong bureaucratic-military oligarchy at the helm of the state which uses its regulatory and controlling powers to mediate the mutually competing and at times conflicting interests of the three dominant classes in the country, while at the same time it protects their specific privileges from potential and actual threats posed by the dispossessed and dominated classes. In this sense, the Pakistan state is not only overdeveloped, but an alien force which wields a disproportionate degree of power over the rest of civil society.[21]

Colonialism also facilitated the rise of the national petty bourgeoisie, the strata that dominated the independence and protest movements in the majority of former colonial countries. It also reinforced existing contradictions within the state and society (e.g. class, race, gender, etc.) that led to the emergence of political forces which would eventually resist structural transformation of the state. The conditions under which the petit bourgeoisie came to power over time could give rise to the Commandist state[22] or the Authoritarian state.[23] The Authoritarian State is:

....the modern, contemporary form of despotic state.

Like all historical forms of the despotic state (feudal, sultanate, bureaucratic, etc.) it seeks to achieve an effective monopoly of sources of power and authority in society for the benefit of the ruling class or elite. The authoritarian state however, in contrast to all other forms of the despotic state, achieves this monopoly by penetrating civil society and transforming its institutions into corporate organizations which act as an extension of the state apparatus. This is the prime characteristic of the authoritarian state, although it differs from one country to another and from one culture to another.[24]

The second criterion of an authoritarian state is that it

penetrates the economic system and attaches it to the state, either by nationalization (for example, in Guyana) or by extending the public sectors to complete state bureaucratic control of economic life. This does not lead to socialism (that is, public ownership of the means of production) as some think, but rather to dependent state capitalism.... What is intended by "dependent state capitalism" is that the state, instead of individual capitalists, takes possession of the social surplus and the surplus value. It is dependent because it enters into unequal economic and political relations with other states, which exposes it to the fluctuations of the capitalist world market, even in the essentials of its existence.[25]

The third characteristic of the 'Authoritarian' state, according to Al NaQeeb, [26]

is that the legitimacy of the system of government in it depends on the use of force (or naked power) and organized terror more than upon traditional legitimacy, and therefore its political system is characterized by the following features in the environment of Third World states in general.

- The absence of governments which represent the interests of the popular masses.

- The absence of meaningful elections.
- The absence of any social organizations independent of the state such as parties, unions, and professional organizations.
- The attainment of power by means of coups, rigged elections or by means other than elections, e.g. force, intimidation, and the organization of terror.
- The legitimacy of the ruling regime based on military force or on violence and intimidation.
- Constitutions annulled or suspended either temporarily or not put into force.
- Civil rights annulled or arbitrarily frozen.
- A high proportion of expenditures monopolized by the army and the apparatus of repression and intimidation.
- The use of the army for purposes of internal security, that is at times other than the emergencies specified in constitutions or appropriate codes.

It is important to stress that the extent to which these characteristics exist within the political systems is determined by the specificity of the societies themselves and the historical conditions that have influenced their development.[27] Petras, for instance, contends that the proliferation of authoritarian and neo-fascist tendencies in the post-colonial and other Third World societies is linked with their essential function to reproduce the conditions to facilitate investment and the operations of metropolitan capital within their territorial spheres.[28]

In the periphery, because of the domination of imperialism over all classes, the national bourgeoisie has been a weak, vacillating, dependent social force, displaying in many instances "little inclination or capacity to develop dynamic national economies...."[29] In the post-colonial period, on the one hand, a number of Third World countries have attempted forms of externally directed industrialization dominated by multinational capital. However,

> externally induced effort limits industrialization in the Third World to particular "moments" of the process whether it be assembly plants, light industry, or capi-

tal goods (without the technical research capacities). Despite the high growth rates which a minority of dependent countries have experienced in recent years, the qualitative aspects, the scope and depth of industrialization have been far from acceptable. [30]

On the other hand, there has been a rejection by some states of the externally directed form of capitalist growth in favour of a national state capitalist model.

> Such a model attempts to devise a different pattern of industrialization linking the various phases of the industrial effort, from technological innovation through assembly, within bounds of the nation state. The key strata initiating and seeming to direct the conversion from neo-colonialism (externally induced expansion) to state capitalism, via evolution, coup, popular uprising, or some combination of the three, are the state sector employees, civil and/or military. This last possibility of capitalist development in the Third World then borrows "socialist forms," political (one-party state, socialist rhetoric, etc.) and economic (state ownership, planning, etc.) to accomplish capitalist ends, namely, the realization of profit within a class society.[31]

Wallerstein's contribution to the understanding of the development of capitalism and the positions of various countries within the "world system" has also been of significant value to the above theoretical discussion.[32] According to Wallerstein,

> ....our capitalist world economy has an aggressive, expansive and efficacious [one]; within a few centuries it encompassed the globe. This is where we are today.[33]

However, his analysis has been characterized by an underlying economism which allows him to assign to the "state a very secondary and sometimes passive role relative to economic forces."[34] In relation to Wallerstein's theory, Simon further states:

> while this may have validity with respect to specific space-time conjunctures, his theoretical analysis generally fails to distinguish the rich texture of interaction

and interrelations between the economy and society mediated by and through different state forms over both time and space.

The assumption of state power by the petit bourgeoisie meant that this stratum was able to take control of state apparatus from the metropolitan bourgeoisie and its local representatives. However, this transition was not designed to turn the state over to the popular masses. Although the petit bourgeoisie had ideas; some self-centred, others idealistic, as a class they lacked the organizational structures required to promote the growth of the economy and safe-guard the advances of the people. They lacked a concept of democracy, and as they embarked on their direction of change, they made hardly any serious attempt to build or democratize the state structures and apparatuses (pertaining to classes, peasantry, marginalized strata) so as to create the conditions for further advance by the people. Their structural limitation may be explained by the fact that, irrespective of the class fraction or stratum that dominated the state apparatuses in the Third World (whether big landowners, merchants, financiers, industrial capitalists or those in control of state power and apparatus), as a group they were still "junior" or "dependent" partners of international capital.[35]

In the Third World, the state particularly, in the post-colonial phase, plays a very important role in the process of production. This development can be attributed to the subordinate and weak nature of social classes that exist. In these formations, there have been some forms of nationalization of important economic areas (e.g. banks, industries, etc.) as well as increasing state intervention in the economy. In addition, the state in the periphery also employs a variety of mechanisms designed to shape the entire development process, including political patronage, discrimination, racism, tax credit and pricing policies, medals and awards, orders, bribery, bullying and relations between state officials and private businessmen.[36] Dale's forceful examination of the world-system theory and its relationship to the state claims that the theory has some limitations.

> The idea that its basic shape is given, by its function in the capitalist world economy, provides a conception of the state which is both limited and distorted,

as well as being excessively instrumentalist, while the associated insistence on the priority of the world system over any national historical or cultural difference does not always seem easy to justify.... What the world-system perspective does is to present a base superstructure model on a world scale, and it shows the strengths and weaknesses of such models.[37]

Gunder Frank in his analysis, argues that capitalist countries of Europe have been exploiting Third World countries since the 16th century and these relations (of exploitation) have continued in a variety of forms until the present day. Because of Gunder Frank's emphasis on capitalist dominance of the entire periphery since the 16th century, his analysis of the state in the Third World follows along similar lines as some of the Third World writers referred to earlier. Thus Gunder Frank sees the state in these societies as structurally weak, dependent, and oppressive.[38]

INDEPENDENT AND NATIONAL LIBERATION MOVEMENTS IN THE PERIPHERY: THE CONTEXT OF THEIR EMERGENCE

Following the division of the world into "the ministries of the great powers" after World War I, the U.S., which was an exception to this policy, "sought to enhance its influence in the international community through an independent strategy."[39] The dominant imperialist powers at that juncture "carved up among themselves the colonial possessions of the defeated nations; prominent among these nations were France, Great Britain, Belgium, the Union of South Africa, Australia, New Zealand and Japan."[40] The reassignment of colonies following the war assumed the form of mandates under Article 22 of the League of Nations Covenant, under which the League "entrusted its international responsibility to govern the territories of particular states."[41] In reality such powers and mandates created the basis for continued exploitation and domination of colonies, for the "new owners were free to integrate the acquired territories as they saw fit."[42]

The October Socialist Revolution in Russia ushered in a new historical era on an international level. It signaled an attempt to emancipate the masses in that part of the world from their material suffering and their conditions of exploitation, oppression and domination. It also was to influence the subsequent struggles against imperialism and independence in colonial societies. In the period between 1924 and 1929 the bourgeoisie in metropolitan centres set out to rationalize production in order to consolidate its dominance. This process involved the introduction of new equipment, plant modernization, and other developments; but it was achieved primarily by such methods as the acute intensification of labour, speed-up of assembly-line and mass operation, sweat-shop system of work, etc. within the capitalist countries. This intensification of production led to substantial increases in the output and hence higher living standards for certain categories of workers. On the other hand,

> "that same rationalization meant physical exhaustion, death from accidents, and loss of their jobs for hundreds of thousands of workers in capitalist countries."[43]

The period 1929-1933 was characterized by world-wide economic collapse. In 1929 "an economic crisis of unprecedented magnitude overtook the capitalist countries,"[44] and its impact was very profound on a global level: industrial overproduction, grave agricultural crisis, financial collapse, bankruptcy among numerous banks, enterprises, and firms, failure of small-business enterprises, massive unemployment, poverty and starvation.[45] The crisis resulted in severe contradictions between the imperialist states and their colonies. It led to a long period of depression which was followed in 1937 by a new economic crisis that ultimately led to the outbreak of the Second World War. The struggle was posed as one against fascism, especially in Germany following the Nazi victory. "The Nazi victory in Germany in 1933, and the unprecedented reign of terror that followed stirred the hitherto slumbering forces of reaction, darkness, chauvinism and war nearly everywhere in the capitalist countries, in some of which these forces were already fighting, to seize the power."[46]

The outbreak of the Second World War was, like that of the First, a product of the capitalist system and its contradictions. The aggressive fascist bloc of Germany, Italy and Japan sought to repatriate the world by force of arms, claiming that they were "cheated out of what was due to them." Of this fascist block, Germany constituted the most dangerous threat to the imperialist States. Hence, a coalition of Western States including Great Britain, France and the United States was formed and later, strengthened by the USSR, they went to war and defeated the Nazis.[47] This war of liberation against fascism powerfully accelerated the anti-colonial struggles in many areas of the world.[48] In respect to the anti-colonial revolution Magdoff writes:

> While colonialism was still on the rise in the interwar years, World War II led not merely to an intensified and better organized nationalism but to a complete reversal of the expansionist trends of the preceding centuries. Now, all large colonial empires began to shrink, to be replaced by a host of new politically independent nations.[49]

Although the defeat of fascism and the outcome of the War created opportunities for Third World states, they nevertheless still had to confront the realities of economic exploitation, colonial domination and racism. The advance of socialism, too, did not lead to a solution of these problems. Socialist transformation also produced a number of contradictions between the socialist states and the periphery in which issues of an economic, political and ideological nature were still part of the relations of domination and dependence. The point to be stressed is that the movement to socialism, though progressive in a number of respects, led to new forms of domination and dependence in the Third World. This was partly due to their structural weakness in the international division of labour. Thus, new military pacts and arrangements and treaties of 'friendship' were established that produced considerable tension over time (e.g., Cuba, Ethiopia, Guyana and the USSR).

THE POST-COLONIAL STATE IN THE CARIBBEAN

The discussion of the state in the Third World to this point has been conducted on a rather abstract and general level, mainly because the object was to advance a number of assumptions relating to the state and state practices in these societies. We now turn specifically to the post-colonial state in the Caribbean. It is important to reiterate a fundamental point in the previous discussion, that is, any rigorous and comprehensive analysis of the state in the periphery of global capitalism must focus on the society's socio-historical, cultural-ideological development and the "underlying structural relations of the society, as this is necessary if its treatment is to transcend the category of a mere political instrument."[50]

"Structural relations" refers to, in addition to those relations mentioned above, class relations, gender relations, relations involving racial contradictions and struggles, social and political movements. Campbell, for instance, makes a critical methodological point which is somewhat relevant to Thomas'. In her research on the Ivory Coast, she makes both general and specific points of interest, contending that there is not an accepted "theory of the post-colonial capitalist state" hence one can offer only provisional solutions. Consequently, the conceptual structure employed should be advanced cautiously with the object of putting forward working hypotheses and posing questions which underscore the "need for a great deal more empirical research before the concepts can be used with any rigour."[51] Therefore, in order to develop a comprehensive analysis of state structures in the Third World during the post-colonial period, it is essential to have a rigorous framework, one that is capable of posing the most pertinent questions that are different "from those which official documents (and more particularly official statistics) are devised to answer."[52] Advancing the point further in relation to the Ivory Coast, Campbell states that:

> the absence of documentation concerning the distribution of national income; the percentage distribution of national income to the highest and lowest quintile, the distribution of access to piped water and electricity, the distribution of landownership particularly in the plantation sector, the absence of such figures is as central a feature of official Ivorian statistics as it is a problem central to the critical analysis of Ivorian society.[53]

This important methodological point regarding the problems

associated with obtaining comprehensive data in the periphery suggests that researchers should be extremely careful when undertaking studies of the state in the periphery. It is in this context, then, that the next analysis, a theoretical examination of the state in the post-colonial Caribbean is done. Some of the arguments which will be used are quite general; however, the purpose is to provide a rigorous and dynamic framework within which the empirical analysis of the study is developed.

In the Caribbean, as in many Third World countries, post World War II developments in the advanced capitalist States of Europe and North America and their effects created material and ideological conditions for the emergence of strong nationalist movements. In response to the struggles, colonial powers

> ceded reforms that, for the first time, introduced multiparty politics in most African [and Caribbean] countries. It was the eve of independence [that] many heralded as the first democratic transition.[54]

Historically, within the Caribbean the colonial state was clearly a non-democratic structure. However, it allowed some democratic movements from the masses to emerge. Following political independence in the 1960s and 1970s, the State structures that became prominent in societies were comparatively small, weak and dependent. In Guyana, however, Forbes Burnham (a former President) expanded and strengthened the unconstitutional State machinery causing it to become anti-democratic, a process which helped to bolster the authoritarian rule of the People's National Congress (PNC).[55]

During the post-colonial phase of economic and social development there has been a tendency towards increasing state control and state intervention not merely within the economy, but also in political and social life.[56] State intervention in the economy resulted from expansion of state institutions and organizations which occurred gradually over the course of development. It should be pointed out that this form of change is not without contradictions and conflicts, given that the peripheral capitalist state is still dominated by international capital, and therefore in many instances does not exercise effective control over the major organs of surplus extraction. In the Caribbean, the continued subordination of the economic and class structure to advanced capitalism results in serious crises; this was especially the case in the 1980s when the advanced capitalist states were experiencing problems themselves.

> The Caribbean is clearly in crisis. If we step back and look at the trajectory of events over the last decade, and study where current trends seem to be leading, the situation can only be described as grim, and the prognosis poor....In these economies unemployment is enormous, there is large out migration and a haemorrhage of skilled people, living standards have declined and human misery increased.[57]

It is correct to argue that the individual societies of the English-speaking Caribbean each have their particular features and have undergone their own experiences. But as Farrell elaborates, this specificity should not obscure some general tendencies among them.

> In almost all countries of the region, the state has come to play a dominant role in economic life. The state has not been just politically dominant. It has not just been key with respect to whatever major investments have taken place, and the direction of drift of the economy. In some of the countries, it has also become big business itself, in terms of direct involvement in the operations of a range of commercial enterprises.[58]

The hegemonic class within the Caribbean in the post colonial era has been the petit bourgeoisie, the stratum which was objectively placed in the position to assume state power following the assumption of constitutional independence in the 1960s and 1970s. But it is this same petit bourgeoisie that would demonstrate over time its class limitations and incapacities of structural transformation. Thus, in explaining the crisis, Farrell contends that

> three things are clear, one is that we have failed. The second is that it is our decisions at governmental level that are primarily to blame. The third is that our future is in the final analysis our responsibility. None of this

is to deny that imperialism or rapacious corporations, or untoward international events or power-hungry trade unionists exist. They do. But enemies, rivals, obstacles and capricious fate are facts of life that one has to live with, overcome or get around. To blame everything imaginable for our failures and exonerate ourselves after two decades and more of independence is silly.[59]

Farrell then concludes that the failures in the Caribbean have been manifested in almost all areas irrespective of the countries' different ideological directions. In demonstrating this point he comments:

First of all the failures have cut right across the ideological spectrum. Burnham's "socialist" Guyana has failed as comprehensively as Bird's "capitalist" Antigua. Eugenia Charles' merchant capitalism has done no better than the Grenadian socialism she so hated. Grenada's socialism itself started out idealistic, self confident and (we can now see with hindsight) even a little self righteous. In less than five years, it soured, degenerated and finally imploded, giving victory to its enemy on a platter, and leaving its people no better off than when it started. Seaga's "born again" capitalism has been no less a disaster for Jamaica than Manley's socialism which is so bitterly derided. Odlam's brief flirtation with socialist rhetoric in St. Lucia ended in confusion and chaos. It proved no better than the capitalism of Compton which preceded it and has now replaced it, and which the first time around ended in similar chaos and confusion.[60]

In explaining further the structural and ideological failures, Farrell makes the important point that explanations for these countries' failures, especially of their economies, cannot be simplistically reduced to their respective sizes or the presence or absence of resources.[61] For, both the micro states as well as the mini ones, those that have poor economic resources for the promotion of socio-economic development, as well as the richer resource-based ones, have been fraught with difficulties that constitute structural barriers to attaining autonomous development.[62]

While internal processes have made their impact, the process of foreign domination undoubtedly has been a major contributory factor of socio-economic backwardness and dependence. With regards to these external forces, Farrell states:

> In terms of foreign domination and even determination of important decisions in the region, we are arguably little less colonized today than we were twenty years ago. Jamaica, Dominica, and Grenada today are simply extravagant forms of a phenomenon that cuts across the entire region. The degree of autonomous response to events has not grown significantly in the last fifteen years.[63]

According to Stone,[64] another scholar of some prominence in the region, after Caribbean states obtained constitutional independence in the 1960s and 1970s, they inherited capitalist-oriented institutions mainly of the Western European type, including constitutions, parliamentary representation, competitive political parties and liberal-democratic political and juridical traditions. Stone also noted that this inherited legacy was bequeathed by the association with Western European colonizers.

> The overwhelming majority of these states have since abandoned that inheritance in favour of military regimes, one-party rule and wide ranging forms of authoritarian rule.[65]

The literature/writings on the post colonial state in the Caribbean reveal a number of fundamental weaknesses. First there is no coherent body of theoretical knowledge on the project with adequate analytical tools. What appears to exist in general are isolated attempts at various moments to grapple with the problem in a serious way. Here the contributions of Thomas, Watson, Munroe, and Rodney stand out. More recently, academics in the region have been attempting to complement these analyses in order to move beyond the constitutional de-colonization and descriptive accounts that have employed "very simplistic forms of periodization."[66]

The majority of Caribbean English-speaking societies at the

end of the colonial period had a set of independent constitutional apparatuses that were shaped and modeled in all essential respects by British imperialist policy and practice. In the early post World War II period the state apparatus was:

> comparatively small in size and highly centralized, and the bureaucracy was not innovative and inefficient. Thus, the state apparatus constituted a poor instrument for directing and regulating economic and social development, though the state was necessarily thrust into this role.[67]

Stephens and Stephens further assert that:

> The new tasks faced by the state in the period after the Second World War, particularly the promotion of industrial and agricultural production, caused an expansion of the functions performed by ministries and the creation of new state agencies in the form of public corporations and regulatory boards.[68]

To elaborate, these writers contend that the structure of the state was conditioned and limited by its link to the metropolis and revealed the characteristics of neo-colonialism.

> Under the colonial administration, the structure of the state was highly centralized, such as to facilitate effective control by the governor in whose hands power was concentrated. After the introduction of self-government, elected ....politicians continued in the tradition of exercising control from above and centralizing power in the hands of ministers and, ultimately, the prime minister. The desire to remain in control stood in contradiction to the need for the creation of new, flexible, and at least partly autonomous state agencies in charge of promoting economic and social development.[69]

Stephens and Stephens have argued fairly forcibly that the colonial legacy of underdevelopment, structural backwardness and exploitation and political and ideological domination was in contradiction with the underlying social realities of the masses' struggles for effective, meaningful changes. Since the metropolitan bourgeoisie was interested in capitalist relations of production expressed through the market system, this means that in many instances for political parties to be seen favourably by the colonial power it was necessary for them to be linked to the private sector.

> The state's capacity to promote and direct economic and social development in the interest of the mass of the people was severely hampered by the close link of both parties to members of the private sector, one manifestation of which was the domination of boards of state agencies by private sector representatives. ... [In instances where] political parties were dependent on private financial contributions and included important capitalist families among their members, many businessmen were appointed as ministers or advisors. As a result of these close links, decision-making in public corporations and agencies increasingly came under the influence of private capital and thus the public sector came to function heavily in the service of private interests.[70]

This increasingly important role of the state in the economy and in socio-political life has been corroborated by other writers. Specifically, Keith and Keith posit that:

> The Jamaican state, for its part, had honed its managerial skills since independence. It became progressively the main procurer of investment capital, inviter of foreign investment, and it emerged as the principal source of capital formation, between 1955 and 1962, the state introduced $420 million in investment; this figure grew to $1.13 billion for the period from 1967 to 1972. After democratic socialism was declared, this role steadily increased. Jamaican capitalists, on the other hand, remained comparatively weak and did not exercise hegemonic power. As class reactions and the activities of the state took on certain anti-imperialist forms, they shared many of the other manifestations of socialism. So did the policies employed by the state. But the crisis was basically a

reaction within capitalism, extraordinary but not enough to initiate a structural transformation of capitalist relations. At work, then, was a process of modification rather than transformation.[71]

The central role of the state has its origin in "peculiar historical circumstances." The Caribbean states, like other Third World countries exposed to colonialism and imperialism, manifest characteristics of and are conditioned by the "peripheral" as distinct from the "advanced" forms of capitalism.[72] Typified by very weak polar classes (that is, the bourgeoisie and proletariat) and sparse capital for development, these economies cannot depend on any developmental impetus that is natural to the antagonisms between powerful capitalist classes and powerful proletariats that are present in advanced economies.[73]

The process of capital accumulation and the regulation of class relations then falls heavily to the state whose role is distinctly different from that of its counterpart in an advanced economy. In peripheral capitalism, the state enjoys significant relevant autonomy, that is, it is less exposed to the constraining power of the poor classes (because of their weakness) though it is no less committed to the continuing existence of capitalism.[74] Hintzen shows that in Guyana, in the late 1960s and 1970s,

> the PNC government utilizing the state apparatuses initiated a set of measures aimed at "controlling" the economic structure of the society. The survival of the PNC depended upon its capacity to satisfy the accumulative claims of the black middle class and the demands of its black supporters for increased job opportunities, for greater job security, and for a larger share of the country's wealth. This necessitated a program of massive state expansion financed through the reallocation of private-sector earnings to the state. Such an emphasis on public sector expansion became evident as soon as the PNC gained.... state control of almost all of the economic activity in the country. This was justified by the regime as the strategy which best assured that developmental goals would be realized. In actuality, it gave to the regime control of the lion's share of the country's resources to be used for the sat-

isfaction of the patronage claims of its black and coloured supporters, particularly the bureaucratic middle class, and perhaps more importantly, to support the system of coercion and control. Together, these underwrite and guarantee the regime survival.[75]

It is evident, given the dependent nature of the ruling classes in the post-colonial societies, that they are unable to promote autonomous capitalist development. Consequently there is widespread unemployment, chronic poverty, economic and social backwardness, uneven development, ideological posturing, and of course, crises. During the post colonial period, because of the peculiar ways in which the state has been linked historically and structurally to the capitalist world economy, the bourgeoisie in the advanced capitalist countries are not required to control directly the state apparatuses. Instead, these weak social classes were given some limited space to "develop" politically and economically, and assume State power through the achievement of constitutional independence. The petit bourgeoisie which consisted of teachers, intellectual academics, professionals, students and others, was the most prominent group in the transition to neo-colonialism. Although they did not constitute the most numerous group in the mass movement, they nevertheless virtually monopolized the articulation of the ideology, the organizational structure and leadership of the movements that were mobilizing for social change. This group was also most prominent in controlling the leading positions in the colonial society when negotiating with the dominant metropolitan power or its local representatives.

The principal role of the petit bourgeoisie was to advance a nationalist and democratic ideology which would not conflict too seriously with the interests of metropolitan capital, but would serve to conceal the specific class contradictions and interests that they represented and hoped to accentuate in the post-colonial period. Thus, the Caribbean petit bourgeoisie was able to exploit the underdeveloped class consciousness of the exploited masses. This was done by appealing for political "unity" despite an ensemble of divergent interests that were being expressed, interests that were not merely reduced to "class," but extended to issues of race, gender, and religion. The petit bourgeoisie advocated "nationalism" and "democracy," drawing (of course) from the struggles conducted in other Third World states (e.g. India, Ghana and others). To a great degree they were 'successful' in achieving these goals even though the metropolitan colonial power still exercised strong influences over those societies which were effectively dominated by imperialism. Instead distorted economic growth was reproduced; this has had serious implications for the society in general but especially for the working people and particularly women who have been experiencing increased poverty. Not being able to effectively meet the needs of the society, many of the states (despite their control over the key resources), became more repressive (in a number of ways) as a way of making sure that the dominant class forces continued to exert their control and power over the state.

This breakdown, though simplistic, does help to provide some basic understanding of the trends in this discussion. However, the existing literature is fundamentally underdeveloped especially when examining the relations of women to the state. Despite these flaws, the analyses that have been produced so far will guide the theoretical discussion which follows. Thomas, the leading critic of the state in the Caribbean, postulates that, in order for the state to be effective, it

> must possess an effective monopoly of physical force over a particular national territory. It also constantly intervenes in other spheres of social life, partly with the intent of reducing the need to resort to the use of its coercive powers directly.... No ruling class wants to or prefers to, rule by force openly and directly. The role of ideology, therefore, is to make force effective by leaving it as an implied last resort, not a first resort of the state. The routine use of force is only resorted to when opinion facing the dominant groups in the state make this a necessity for their own survival. Such conjunctures I define as crises of the regimes in power, and possibly (depending on the circumstances) as crises of the state and society itself.[76]

In addition, although the state, emerged historically as a class institution in the Caribbean, this does not mean that it must be seen as a simple or automatic instrument of the ruling class.[77]

Thomas adds:

> In the Caribbean there are several reasons for this. One is that the class origins of the personnel who run the state machinery are not necessarily the same as those of the ruling class. Another is that the ruling class has not been historically a homogeneous group. Many contending factions exist, with the result that there is no simple, except for the simple-minded, determination of the general interest of the ruling class. Indeed the state often has acted as a mediating factor in the contentions of these various factions of the ruling class, thereby exhibiting elements of independence in relations to the social basis.[78]

Another point of emphasis in Thomas' analysis is that the state is a historical materialist category. This means that any serious analyses of the state must concentrate on its social and material bases in the context of its historical development.[79] Finally "at this historical conjuncture a central feature of the state is the role of representative/constitutional/political democracy in its functioning."[80]

Although Thomas must be complimented for undertaking such an interesting project, his analysis has been conducted primarily on the economic level, though references have been made on political questions. Thomas' perspective or framework must, therefore, be expanded in order to adequately deal with the issues and problems facing women. The literature on the state in the region for the most part has been dominated by men's writings and thus lacks a comprehensive, critical understanding of the social realities of women's lives. In order to obtain this perspective, it is important that women's own perceptions and understanding of their conditions of material, social and personal life be given central importance similar to that which has been attributed to men's struggles. Thus, because the struggles and concerns of women, particularly those who are the most marginalized (economically, politically, culturally, ideologically, socially powerless on the basis of gender), must be considered. The literature on the state examined to this point generally still reflects the hierarchical tendencies that have dominated the social formations from slavery through colonial times and to the present. This is succinctly articulated by Wolff who stated that:

> We must recognize that the majority of studies of "Third World" cultures have described the experiences of men at the expense of those women. As in every other intellectual and academic pursuit until recently, women have remained more or less invisible as a result of gender-biased investigations.[81]

The above points serve to indicate that researchers have to be extremely careful when undertaking studies of the state and the social relations within it in the Third World. This observation is even more critical, as already pointed out, when discussing women's conditions of existence in these societies. To take cognizance of this fact, it is important to incorporate a feminist perspective into the discussion of the societies in question their cultural relations and global connections. For it will be observed that these relations and practices (economic, political, ideological, institutional) are connected to and intertwined with issues of the family, social relations of gender, sexuality, the domestic sphere, and with the sexual division of labour, and therefore must be addressed within this context, within the social sciences in general and, for this purpose, sociology in particular. In other words,

> ... we must be prepared to investigate the interrelations of public and private, of the economy and the domestic, of male and female roles, and of ideologies, of work and politics and ideologies of gender in our attempt to theorize the global dimensions of culture and society.[82]

The next chapter, which is a review of the available literature on women and the Caribbean state, will address these issues with more seriousness as well as with appropriate theoretical tools.

Notes

1. Ben Crow *Survival and Change in the Third World*. London: Polity Press, 1988: 340.
2. Ibid.
3. Michel-Rolph Trouillot " *Haiti: State against Nation: The origins and legacy of Duvalierism.*" New York: Monthly Review Press,

      1990: 22-23.
4.   Ibid.
5.   Anton L Allahar *Sociology and the Periphery: Theories and Issue,* Toronto: Garamond Press, 1989: 110-111.
6.   see Richard Harris and Carlos M Milas (eds.). *Nicaragua A Revolution Under Seige.*: Zed Books Ltd., 1985:10-32.
7.   Michael W Foley and Thomas F. Love (eds.) *State, Capital and Rural Society.* Boulder: Westview Press Inc., 1989:40.
8.   Hamza Alavi "The State in Post-Colonial Societies: Pakistan and Bangladesh." *New Left Review* 74: (1972):59-81.
9.   Ibid.
10. David Simon *Cities, Capital and Development.* London: Belhaven Press, 1992:8-9.
11. Ibid.
12. see James Cypher *State and Capital in Mexico-Development Policy since 1940.* Boulder: Westview Press, Inc., 1990:7 .
13. Ibid.:35-36.
14. Ibid.:36-37.
15. Ibid.
16. Ian Roxborough *Theories of Underdevelopment.* London: Macmillian, 1979:123.
17. Barbara Stalling *Class Conflict and Economic Development in Chile 1973-1985.* :Stanford University Press, 1978:15-16.
18. Fawzy Mansour *The Arab World: Nation State and Democracy.*: Zed Press, 1992 :89-90.
19. Ibid.
20. Hassan N Gardezi. *A Reexamination of the Social Political History of Pakistan.*: New York: Edwin Meller Press, Lewiston, 1990: 90.
21. Ibid.
22. see Horace Campbell "The Commandist State in Uganda." Political Research in Progress Seminar Paper: University of Sussex, 1977.
23. see CY. Thomas. "The Authoritarian State in Caribbean Societies" *The State in Caribbean Societies.* ed.), Omar Davies: University of the West Indies, Mona 1986:63; Al-NaQeeb (1990): 99-100.
24. Kladoum Hassan Al-NaQeeb, *Society and State in the Gulf and Arab Peninsula: A Different Perspective*, London: Routledge and Kegan Paul, 1990:99-100.
25. Ibid.:100.
26. Ibid.:100-101.
27. Ibid.:101.
28. See Hassan N Gardezi.: 1991: 90.
29. James Petras *Critical Perspectives on Imperialism and Social Classes in the Third World.* New York: Monthly Review Press,

1978:84.
30. Ibid.:85.
31. Ibid.:86.
32 See Immanuel Wallerstein "The State and Social Transformation" *Politics and Society* 1: 1971, 1980, 1990.
33. Immanuel Wallerstein "World System Versus World Systems: A Critique" *Critique of Anthropology* 2: 1974: 189-194.
34 David Simon *Cities, Capital and Development* : Belhaven Press, 1992:6.
35. see Henry Berstein, Ben Crow and Mary Thorpe, et al (eds.). *Survival and Change in the Third World*. London: Polity Press, 1988.
36. Nigel Harris *The End of the Third World*. London: I.B. Tauris & Co. Ltd., 1986: 41-42.
37. Roger Dale "Nation State and International Systems: the World System Perspective." G. McLenor, D. Held, and S. Hall, (eds.). *The Ideas of the Modern State*. Milton Keynes: the Open University Press, 1984:205-206.
38. Andre Gunder Frank "The Development of Underdevelopment" (eds.) James D. Andre Gunder Frank, and Dale L. Johnson. *Dependence and Underdevelopment*: Latin America's Political Economy: New York:Anchor Books, Doubleday & Company Inc. 1972: 3-17.
39. Harry Magdoff *Imperialism: from the Colonial Age to the Present*. New York: Monthly Review Press, 1978:62.
40. Ibid.:63.
41. Ibid.
42. Ibid.
43. AZ. Manfred. (ed.). *A Short History of the World*. Moscow: Progress Books, 1974:13.
44. Ibid:134.
45. Ibid.
46. Ibid.: 140-42.
47. Ibid.:276.
48. R.P. Dutt. *The Crisis of Britain and the British Empire*. London: Lawrence and Wishart, 1953:92; see also H. Magdoff: 1978.
49. Ibid.: 67.
50. Clive Thomas "The Authoritarian State in Caribbean Societies."(ed.) Omar Davies, *The State in Caribbean Society*, Mona, Jamaica: University of the West Indies, Department of Economics, 1986, Monograph 2:63.
51. Bonnie Campbell "The Ivory Coast." (ed.), John Dunn *West African States: Failure and Promise*.: Cambridge University Press, 1987:66.
52 Ibid.:66.

53. Thomas: 1986:63.
54. Mahmood Mamdani "Democratic Theory and Democratic Struggles." *Dissent* :Summer, 1992:313.
55. Clive Thomas: 1986:2.
56. R Nettleford. "Chairman's Introductory Remarks." (ed.) Omar Davies, *The State in Caribbean Society*, Mona, Jamaica:University of the West Indies, Department of Economics, 1986, Monograph 2:3.
57. Trevor Farrel "The Caribbean State and its Role in Economic Management." (ed.) Omar Davies, *The State in Caribbean Society*, Mona, Jamaica: University of the West Indies, Department of Economics, 1986, Monograph :6.
58. Ibid.:9.
59. Ibid.:7.
60. Ibid.:8.
61. Ibid.:9.
62. Ibid.:8-9.
63. Ibid.:9.
64. Carl Stone "Democracy and the State: The Case of Jamaica." (ed.), Omar Davies, *The State in Caribbean Society*. Mona, Jamaica: University of the West Indies, Department of Economics, 1986, Monograph 2.:90.
65. Ibid.
66. see Patrick Emmanuel, 1988; Clive Thomas, 1984 and 1988; Walter Rodney, 1974; 1980.
67. Evelyn Huber Stephens and John D Stephens. *Democratic Socialism in Jamaica*: Macmillian, 1986:39.
68. Ibid.
69. Ibid.:39.
70. Ibid.:41.
71. Nelson W Keith and Novelle Z. Keith. *The Social Origins of Democratic Socialism in Jamaica*. Philadelphia: Temple University Press, 1992:30.
72. Ibid.:39.
73. Ibid.
74. Ibid.
75. Percy Hintzen *The Cost of Regime Survival: Racial Mobilization, Elite Domination and Control of the State in Guyana and Trinidad*. Cambridge: Cambridge University Press, 1989:157-161.
76. Clive Thomas (1986):63.
77. Ibid.
78. Ibid.:63-64.
79. Ibid.:64.
80. Ibid.

81. James Wolff "The Global and the Specific: Reconciling Conflicting Theories of Culture." *Culture, Globalization and World System*, (ed.) Anthony D. King, Binghampton: Department of Art History, State University of New York, 1991: 169.

82. Ibid.:170.

CHAPTER 3

WOMEN AND THE CARIBBEAN STATE

This chapter attempts to examine the ways in which the post colonial state[1] in the English-speaking Caribbean has been analyzed in relation to gender, class, and race with special emphasis on women and the State. It assesses the historical and current literature on Caribbean women in order to examine how their experiences have been represented. Finally, it looks at reasons why Caribbean women have been misrepresented and made "invisible" despite their important historical contributions and sociological functions in their societies. Caribbean women, according to Pulsipher, were historically involved in multifaceted roles as

> agricultural laborers, in the organization of domestic life, with material culture, family organization, child bearing customs, value systems, gender relations, food production and distribution.[2]

The objective of this chapter is to selectively review of the literature on the post colonial state and women in the Caribbean, seeking to illustrate common themes and issues which lead to the theoretical and methodological framework for the study. Recent Caribbean feminist discourse on the state in the Caribbean will be examined for adequacy of explanation of the underlying structural realities within these societies.

Within recent times, there has been a growing recognition amongst Caribbean social scientists and researchers of the importance of women's contributions to, at various levels, the region's realities.[3] Here as previously mentioned, women's own perceptions and understanding of their conditions of material, social and personal life are of fundamental importance in any consideration of their historical position and roles within these societies and in relation to the state. Brereton, a Caribbean historian, in discussing the "General Problems and Issues in Studying the History of Women," asserts that

> since the late 1960s it has been very generally recognized that women have been invisible in the conventional historical record, they have been "hidden from history".... In conventional history; the only history up to about 60 years ago and still in the popular perception the real, orthodox, mainstream history - women are simply not there, except for the odd ruling woman when she cannot be ignored ("women at the top"). Here we have half of "mankind" with no history apparently worth recording. The neglect and ignorance of women in history were almost total.[4]

Brereton attributed the 'neglect and ignorance' partly to the way in which historical questions were posed and issues were described and/or analyzed:

> at the risk of over simplification, history was conventionally defined as the ideas and action of male members of the ruling classes of past societies. It was about government, state building, war, formal institutions, founding official religions, mastering the environment; all activities in which the male elites believed that women's roles were insignificant, or at best supportive only... The exclusion of women from conventional history thus reflected systems of gender oppression and in turn reinforced them by encouraging the defi-

nition of women as the "Other," the passive, there but not there, never the makers and movers of history.[5]

Moving from more general formulations to the specific features of Caribbean historical realities and women's relationship to them, Brereton advances a number of salient points. First, she attempts to develop a feminist approach to understanding gender issues as they have developed historically. Brereton suggests that, despite the complex nature of the subject,

> [h]istorians of the Caribbean need to bring this kind of conceptual perspective to their work, so that female roles and gender systems can be inserted into the historical record.... work has already begun, though only recently, and here I want only to suggest lines of investigation to develop or to continue.[6]

This progressive approach to research advocated by Brereton follows closely the perspective of Joan Scott who articulates:

> the position of gender concerns (or sexual differences) should be incorporated as a category of historical analysis in the historian's analytical tool-box in order to facilitate a genuine rewriting of history.[7]

Second, in terms of research projects on Caribbean women, Brereton noted that an understanding of slavery and its effects on women provides "a promising start," for it allows an examination of the role of women within the slave-based economy (i.e. as agricultural workers and producers), their experience of family life, and their role in resistance to slavery.[8] However, since Caribbean slave material sources are not very rich and the evidence for conducting such an analysis is "scanty, confusing, ambivalent and often downright misleading; in some areas it may well be simply non-existent...",[9] important questions must be raised and an appropriate theoretical perspective for answering them must be formulated so that policies, programmes and services for women can be developed and implemented.

The third point that Brereton mentioned is also of fundamental importance because it relates to an issue which, historically, has been part of the colonial and imperialist systems of domination, that is, the production and reproduction of source materials. Referring to research on the history of Indo-Caribbean women, an area that is underdeveloped, this feminist scholar concludes that the available sources

> are scattered and inadequate, especially as the bulk of the primary materials, written by officials, planters and Churchmen, are imbued with both racism and sexism.[10]

This point seems to be consistent with the one made by Campbell earlier. The experiences of both Afro-and Indo-Caribbean women have shown that at the end of the slave and indentured periods many of them who entered into wage labor on the sugar estates eventually withdrew from these conditions of production

> in order to become peasant producers and marketers. This was no retreat to the home for them.... The peasant woman was an integral part of the household economy, combining production (crops and livestock) and marketing with childcare and housework.[11]

The reasons for the decline of female participation in the plantation labor force between the late nineteenth century and the early 1940s continues to be debated. Did women voluntarily withdraw their labor so that they could concentrate on subsistence agriculture and familial ties? Or was it an involuntary response to the reproductive and productive requirements of the colonial economy? The chronic poverty experienced by the working class during this period seems to indicate that it was, to a great degree, the latter; "due to retrenchment and a lack of sufficient 'women's jobs'"[12] It is important to note that

> women who were usually unskilled and defined as less productive laborers would always be vulnerable to retrenchment when industries were depressed, mechanization had changed employment needs, and men were available. The official attitude was to see declining female participation in the paid labor force as desirable, but working class women in the Caribbean had always seen their proper role as multiple and flexible, as provider, mother and sometimes wife. When fewer could secure wage work, this must have affected

their control of income, the diet and health of themselves and their children, their fertility and their sense
of self worth ...[13]

Caribbean societies are essentially patriarchal societies despite
the aborted efforts at socialist transformation, for example in
Grenada. "Patriarchy" refers to a structure of social relationships
through which men systematically exploit women, one that produces and reproduces the conditions for male domination and
female subordination. It is a structural phenomenon and has
equal importance to other structural features of these societies
such as racism and dependency. Since patriarchy does not constitute a set of specific and absolute relationships, the forms that
it takes vary between societies. In the Caribbean, however, there
have been certain common and general tendencies that center
around women's conditions of work and existence, their position
within the colonial and post-colonial divisions of labor, domestic
labor, male violence and sexuality.

Patriarchal social structures have existed in the Caribbean for
centuries. Gender divisions constitute one of the major divisions
in the context of the region's development. However, in relative
terms, issues relating to gender (especially when they have to do
with patriarchal dominance) continue to be inadequately formulated and addressed in the theoretical literature. Issues affecting
women are often either neglected or completely ignored. The literature on the state, as is evident from the early discussion in this
chapter, still reflects this fundamental theoretical and methodological weakness, the relegating of women and their struggles
to insignificance, and the inadequate treatment of their conditions
of existence. This weakness may have partly resulted from the
complex nature of the societies in question as well as from the
effects of a colonial domination on the subjects themselves.
Whatever the explanation, this situation is unacceptable. Wiltshire-Brodber asserts that

> the Caribbean gender issue cannot be divorced from
> the fact that Caribbean men and women cannot
> respect and value each other if as people they do not
> respect and value themselves.[14]

In order to discuss issues related to the lives of women, their identities and conditions of existence in societies such as Barbados, Grenada and the Caribbean or Latin America, it is necessary to have some understanding of historical relations (such as colonial conquest, slavery, neocolonialism) and how these impacted on women of different racial and socio-economic classes.[15]

Therefore, when we examine the social relations of women to the state and the effects of state policies and practices on them, the analysis itself has to encompass and contextualize many important elements which go beyond economic and political structures and practices notwithstanding their crucial importance. It is important to take note of, and examine such factors as reproductive responsibilities, gender, social and cultural identities and, according to Vargas,

> images and practices that shape everyday behavior, symbolism and place in political culture. In other words, we are looking also at (self) representation of gendered politics and protest (however small these might be), and how identities are forged within certain "technologies" of racism and gender.[16]

In the Caribbean in general, and specifically in relation to Barbados and Grenada, it is necessary to examine the specific features of the economy and society, the state and class relations, the array of complex and contradictory processes and women's relationship to these. For it becomes obvious that in numerous accounts of these societies' socio-economic, political and cultural-ideological developments, many aspects pertaining to women's lives and struggles are glossed over, concealed, ignored, trivialized or marginalized.

Theories of women's conditions of existence and struggle are formulated in rather general terms in the literature reviewed. "Women's" issues are not addressed in a rigorous manner. Analysts tend to relegate gender issues to a secondary position, even in seemingly progressive discourses. For instance, Marxist and socialist scholars mainly tend to address class relations and class struggles (which are regarded as indispensable) to transform oppressive and exploitative social relations. As illustrated in the previous discussion on the state in the periphery (including the Caribbean) some progress has been made in this respect. However, in the context of women's historical development in the region, problems concerning gender may have had or continued to have their own unique characteristics and specific conditions of emergence and existence which cannot be merely reduced to class (production) relations.

Therefore, in pursuing their lines of investigation, researchers on/in the region have to be sensitive to the fact that there are gender specific issues in colonial and post-colonial societies.

Incorporating these issues into a Marxist, socialist or feminist framework in a simplistic, or mechanistic or reductionist manner, without carefully locating their uniqueness or particular aspects, may serve to mask the specific norms, values and class interests that may be dominating such analyses. Class relations constitute one aspect of social relations, albeit a critically important one. However, with respect to women's oppression, domination, exploitation and dependence, it is necessary to advance a wider perspective, one which is capable of viewing women's oppression within a wider context.[17]

There is a need, in analyzing women's inferior position in society to go beyond the exploitation of domestic labor or the contradictions between capital and labor for "where female disadvantage is identified more generally, it is readily categorized as an instance of patriarchy."[18] In social theory a number of stages of women's oppression have been identified. Even though the emphasis has been on the advanced capitalist countries, many of the points mentioned have relevance to Caribbean development. Walby argues that gender analysis has gone through four stages, presumably as an academic response to the discussions of feminism originating in the late 1960s.[19] The first stage focused on

> how women had been neglected or excluded from studies altogether. In sociology, this has been especially noted in stratification theory, where the study of class relations had been usually confined to males. Otherwise women had been "hidden from history."[20]

Walby, in referring to the second stage, points out that this neglect of women should be used to expose the theoretical and empirical fallacies which become glaringly transparent on the basis of the first stage.

In the theory of class it becomes possible to demand stratification for women and to question whether a wife adopts the class mantle of her husband, and it can even be proposed that women constitute a separate class. In history, the role of women in community and other struggles come to the fore.[21]

The third stage in the development of women's studies is one in

which models or analyses of women are added on to those for men, to fill the gender vacuum that has long been discovered alongside the orthodoxy. Here there are separate models of women in the labor market and separate histories and sociologies of women, and an opening up of the "private" as opposed to the "public."[22]

Finally, Walby asserts that the importance of the fourth and current stage is

recognizing, and attempting to move beyond, the unsatisfactory analytical creation of a dualism in the models of gender relations, one model for men which might have previously been presumed to have been sufficient despite having implicitly excluded women and, in reaction against this, a separate set of models for women. Consequently integration is sought between the two sorts of models so that the relative position and role of men and women are understood simultaneously and symbiotically.[23]

Although this theoretical insight by Walby is to be appreciated for periodizing women's studies into stages, it

is undoubtedly too stylized and forced for general application. It is totally inappropriate, for example, for psychology and anthropology where, however satisfactory and accurately, women long occupied a central role. The same is also obviously true for much of the content of cultural studies. Consequently, the impact of a new wave of feminism upon them has been entirely different.[24]

To pose the question of women's struggles, development and gender identity in the context of Latin American and Third World development, for Vargas

> also means turning our view to the path of conquest, of colonization; to how peasant women have been forced into submission; to the slavery of black women; to the historically rooted isolation of middle class women to the effects of these and other crises in women's lives, to the strong presence of the traditional Catholic Church (and other denominations) in the lives of many women. In sum, to the traces each and all these experiences leave upon the minds and bodies of this heterogeneous category of women.[25]

Research on gender issues, especially those relating to political protest in the Caribbean and Latin America, to a great degree has emphasized those factors which Westwood and Radcliffe have referred to as "externalities." However, a more comprehensive view of women necessitates further analysis that would consider the "internalities" as well. These two aspects of research have been summarized in the following manner:

> ....research has tended to focus particularly on the "externalities" of political protest.... [however, it is important] to contextualize women's protest not only in terms of pre-existing political organizations, socioeconomic structures and reproductive responsibilities, but also to uncover some of the 'internalities' of political protest, like gender and political identities, images and practices that shape everyday behavior, symbolism and place in political culture. In other words, we are looking also at (self) representation of gendered politics and protest, and how identities are forged within certain "technologies" of racism and gender.[26]

Specifically in relation to the Caribbean, it is important to examine particular features of the economic structures and societies especially for the purpose of the study in relation to Barbados and Grenada. Morrissey, for instance, has pointed out that

> the most meaningful task of those engaged in histor-

ical comparison is the construction of sufficiently discrete and specific analytical categories to account for the unique experiences of social groups.[27]

Morrissey further contends that despite the efforts made by various researchers to provide different explanations of the historical and cultural realities of Caribbean women's lives during slavery, the fact remains that

> Caribbean bondwomen were relatively powerless in their communities and [were victimized] through several forms of inequality and exploitation.[28]

"Dependency" theories and "world system" perspectives have attempted to explain the relationship between the advanced capitalist countries and the dominated States of the Third World. Within the dependency perspectives though, Morrissey asserts that:

> non-capitalist regions and workers in the non-wage sector, in particular women, were largely ignored. Yet many questions about the underdevelopment of Caribbean economies in the mid and late nineteenth century go back to the slave era and involve women's role in production and reproduction.... [therefore] any such study of....women reflects the paradox, the twists and turns of social relations endemic to Third World capitalism and the articulation with non-capitalist social and economic systems.[29]

The history of women in the Caribbean will reveal and underscore a very important fact, that they were in

> a constant, dynamic struggle with men, both slave and free, over the foundations of their social experiences.... [Furthermore] females' lack of access to skilled agricultural work diminished their social status and authority, and gender became an increasingly salient expression of stratification within communities of Caribbean slaves and among free men and women.[30]

Although there have been instances in the anti-colonial struggles when women as well as men resisted colonial forms of domination, subordination and imperialism, the underlying reality was that women functioned in a set of uneven social relations dominated by men. These structural relations, in fact, continue to exist despite some progress made by women.

Given the importance of slavery as an economic and social system throughout the English-speaking Caribbean, any serious study of the exploitation and domination of women requires an understanding of the underlying social relations of enslavement. Indeed, it is through the imposition of slave relations on the communal social structures of the indigenous peoples, that the conditions for the introduction and the reproduction of private property forms of commodity production were established. Morrissey has already shown that the basis for women's exploitation, their powerlessness and inequality, was to be sought in the slave conditions prevalent in these societies. Green, a Caribbean feminist writer, corroborates some of the assertions that Morrissey makes in addition to emphasizing the dominant historical and ideological tendencies which permeated men's perception of, and writings on, Caribbean slave women. Reformulating assumptions that characterized the discourse of Adam Smith, and others long after him, she writes:

> In 1776 Adam Smith wrote, in an authoritative and proprietary voice: "Among our slaves in the West Indies there is no such thing as a lasting union. The female slaves are all prostitutes and suffer no degradation by it." Thus, and in a multitude of other ways.... did the alleged "culture" of the oppressed come to constitute a subterranean cesspool in which ruling whites disposed of and concealed their refusal of culpability, conferring it instead upon their victims as the latter's "native heritage."[31]

While Smith's overt racism and contempt for Black women cannot be obscured or denied from the above comments, it is important to mention that similar assumptions form part of the discourse on women and slavery long after the period for which Smith gained his socio-economic reputation with his *Wealth of Nations.* Patterson, a Black Caribbean-born sociologist, writing in more recent times, seems to be wedded in some respects to views on black women that are similar to Smith's. He wrote that:

> Slaves [in the West Indies] mated promiscuously and
> sometimes in outright prostitution; in sporadic unions;
> in relatively stable unions; in quasi-polygamous
> unions; and rarely, in marriage.... Promiscuity was
> common, especially among the women....(Emphasis
> added).[32]

To demonstrate that the above quotation from Patterson was not
an isolated reference taken out of context, Green shows that his
thinking with respect to Black women could be elicited from
some of his other observations and writings in which he attempts
to rationalize Black men's domination of Black women. Patterson reasons (and condones) that the negative behavior of Black
men to Black women is an expressed frustration of their experiences of exploitation and humiliation by white patriarchal relations,

> ....observe that the compensatory behavior on the
> part of Black men in the face of their own humiliation,
> domination and objectification of Black women,
> sometimes seeing conquest of Black women as a
> means through which they could repair their wounded
> pride.[33]

Patterson seems to be rationalizing the fact that Black men,
given the abuse to which they themselves were subjected under
the dominance of Europeans, sought to "compensate" for their
exploitation and domination by relating to women as objects to
"conquer." In other words,

> ....wounded Black men as the primary casualty of
> White Patriarchy; non-intellectual Black women (Black
> female bodies) as the sensuous medium (or objects?)
> of a nonpuritanical (orgiastic?) Caribbean culture.[34]

This mode of reasoning, according to Green, suggests "the
misogyny inherent in Patterson's entire repertoire of ideas."[35]
Patterson, unlike Garvey, discredits and minimizes the struggles
of women. However, although Green would credit Garvey as an
anti-colonial and anti-racist champion of women's leadership
and participation in the UNIA (United Negro Improvement Asso-

ciation) in a way that no other nationalist leader had before, he nonetheless

> upheld with reverence the notion of the woman as the homemaker, culture bearer and as someone who intrinsically carried the memory of the race.[36]

Green's analysis is rigorous in that she brings to the fore, men's conception and understanding of women's position historically in Caribbean societies. She was able to demonstrate the theoretical weakness across time in their analysis when they refer to women:

> What Adam Smith, Orlando Patterson, B.W. Higman and Marcus Garvey all have in common, in spite of the critical divisions of race, class and ideology which separates them, is that, as men, they have been privileged makers of history, and in their accounts or praxes, women have figured, to varying degrees, as objects or reflections of male subjects, the raw material of male invention. Note that it is not my intention to trivialize the difference between these men.

Green, following her critique of these important men, advances an alternative position which she feels will serve her undertaking well. She attempts, therefore,

> .... not just to "factor women in" but also to begin to rewrite West Indian/Caribbean history from the point of view of Black women, specifically during the period of slavery, and to do so through a critique of masculinist interpretations and manipulation of the historical data.[37]

To this end, she utilizes two important concepts that have analytical status to focus on those areas of women's lives which men either intentionally or unintentionally seem to miss, namely, "the combined activities of goods-production and human-reproduction"[38] (i.e. production and reproduction). Clarifying these concepts, Green makes the following argument:

> The first thing that strikes one about the origins of Afro-Caribbean women's economic role is the extent

to which their lives as slaves were defined by the imperatives of extra-domestic, gang-based field production of export staples for an "alien" class and "alien" community of consumers. Where most women's histories appear to "begin" with the family or domestic-based re/production and move outwards extra-domestically or further inwards towards an inner sanctum of reproductive specialization, privacy and seclusion or isolation, Afro-Caribbean women begin their history as coerced, "public" laborers alienated from their own bodies and "birthright" in a system based on reproductive artificiality. Thereafter, they appear to move back and forth between alienated production or service for others and attempts to restore or reconstitute, often single handedly, that birthright.[39]

Slave society, insofar as it has affected women and in terms of its connection to international capitalism, has a number of important features which may be summarized along these lines:[40]

a. unremitting field labor; sexual division of labor. Women performed dual roles as field laborers and domestic workers but were generally denied the more high skilled slave occupations such as technicians in the factory, the plantations artisans or craftsmen, and the head drivers in the field;

b. workers or breeders; reproductive coercion. Here it should be mentioned that slave fertility was notoriously low with fifty percent of the population being childless; sometimes interpreted as an anti-natalist policy by the plantation owners who viewed the women as "producers" rather than "reproducers";

c. women were regarded as sex objects; they were denied spousal, parental and family rights ("the sexual exploitation of slave women by white men was very high in the Caribbean"[41]). Black slave men were discouraged from forming permanent unions; and therefore men were denied parental and family rights. This meant that women were left alone to perform these multiple roles;

d. autonomy and resistance; provision grounds; Sunday markets and cultural reconstitution.[42]

In relation to this final feature, Green asserts that

> Slave women must be understood not just as victims but as historical subjects and social agents who placed certain limits on assault on their dignity and the level of humiliation they were prepared to endure, who fought back, who refused to cooperate with planter-class designs and directives, who participated in efforts to bring down the system, who asserted their own identities and cultural mores, and who seized hold of opportunities offered by the system to widen and deepen their sphere of entitlement, agency and autonomy.[43]

The history of women has received scant attention from social historians in the region. Because of this gap in the historical documents, a comprehensive and accurate analysis of the social realities of the region is severely restricted generally. Thus, Tucker's view is

> if we fail to comprehend women's activities, we fail to come to terms with the activities and institutions of most women and men alike.[44]

She further identifies two tasks for the social analyst seeking to provide a dynamic and rigorous analysis of these societies in question. First,

> we need to develop a broad understanding that can encompass the rhythms and features of the indigenous society as well as the patterns of European penetration.[45]

Secondly, with respect to specific and concrete analysis, one

> must continue to conduct the focused studies that can help us understand how people lived during the period.[46]

Thus, there is a dialectical relationship between the two approaches to the historical study of society, women and, more broadly, the relations of gender:

> while the broad understanding provides the frame-

work within which we can orient our work and learn to ask significant questions, the focused studies will help test and refine our broad understanding.[47]

In focusing on women's development in the region with social science tools, one has to be concerned not only with how women experienced the "big changes" dominated by European capital but also with how they themselves contributed to them either directly or indirectly. In other words,

[i]t is the way people lived these changes; the way they perceived, struggles against, accommodated, or actively encouraged them; that gives these changes their content as well as their historical meaning.[48]

There must be a connection between the macro and micro aspects of development in any socio-historical perspective of women, specifically Caribbean women, because the

"macro" and "micro" form a seamless whole: the major historical developments of the modern period are inextricably tied up with the multitude of ways in which people, as individuals, families, classes, and genders, made these developments possible.[49]

The subordinate position of women in Caribbean society and in relation to the State structures is not an accidental one for the effects of colonialism were profound indeed.

Colonial power relations find expression in words as much as in actions. Relations of power are embedded in Europeans colonial discourses, which create hierarchies and typologies that establish difference, render silent, exclude or incorporate indigenous Others .... Relations between colonizer and colonized are relations of dominance, subjugation, oppression, control, transformation.[50]

In concluding this part of the discussion, it is appropriate to make some pertinent observations which are interrelated in fundamental aspects. For the most part, it has been evident that attempts by social researchers to examine the position of women within Caribbean social formations have been articulated with social scientific categories and modes of explanation.

For example, some of the theories and analyses, particularly those by men have been characterized by problems, either because of the propensity to be too simplistic about very complex structures and social relations, or because the discourses were conducted within the structure of patriarchal relations and with masculinist ideology. In the first instance, the contributions tend to be too descriptive and lack any explanatory or interpretive power. In situations where attempts have been made to provide casual explanations, seeking to understand how and why women's relation to the State has taken on such forms, analyses have not been very clear, and, for the most part, have assumed a particular ideological position.

Within more recent times, however, there has been a decisive shift in the terms of the discussion with the intervention of "Caribbean feminists or 'womanist' historians"[51] and Third World social scientists. Some of these discussions have been very useful at the theoretical, methodological and empirical levels. A number of these perspectives are working within the historical materialist tradition, refining and extending it in order to explain the concrete realities in these societies. However, as Reddock has asserted:

> ....in spite of the steady increase in published and unpublished material, we are continually astounded by how much is still unknown, unexplored and unresearched.[52]

Contributions of "Third World" feminists to the literature on the state, though not extensive, have focused on some of the critical issues confronting women; especially those women in the periphery who are the most exploited and oppressed by, and subordinated to, the relations of peripheral capitalism dominated by men. For example, some exciting contemporary research studies and writings have been done in the areas of women's organizing, food production, higglering, domestic and agricultural labor.[53]

It is fair to say that from the interest shown thus far in the discussions on the realities and conditions of the masses of women in these societies, some progress has been made. However, this fact should in no way prevent us from pointing out some of the theoretical weaknesses and inadequacies in the literature. From the arguments advanced by a number of feminist writers (some of whom have strongly identified with and integrated themselves into the struggles and forms of resistance of the masses of women in the Third World) it appears that they have recognized the importance of analyzing their struggles with rigorous theoretical tools. This means that these tools should be able to get to the essence of the problems confronting women in important areas of their socio-economic, political, cultural, ideological and personal lives. Furthermore, they should be able to help women in the dominated and dependent periphery to extricate themselves from those experiences that have historically and geographically kept them, as a group, in subordinate, exploitative and oppressive relations. These relations are economically, politically and psychologically binding and have systematically excluded women from meaningful and effective interventions and participation in the processes and conditions that would lead to social and structural transformation. Above all, more attention and importance must be given to those women who have experienced and are actually experiencing the variety and forms of exploitation in their lives and struggles.[54]

Of course, to accomplish this goal, women would have to continue struggling in these societies, where to a great extent they are regarded as the "other," in order to obtain the autonomous base which would enable them to move beyond their isolation, individualization, and subordination, and lead to the development of a collective consciousness that will help to change their own realities.[55]

Finally, it is evident, given the complexity of the region, that further investigation of a socio-economic, historical, and sociological nature into the entire question of women's conditions of existence is in order. For until such scholarship is undertaken more extensively and rigorously, it will be impossible to specify the changing characteristics of the state and its relationship to the fundamental issues concerning women. The next task of the study or research, therefore, is to connect the theoretical insights derived from this chapter to a historical and contemporary examination of the Caribbean State, the health care system and women.

The theory of the post-colonial state in the Caribbean provided a useful framework in which the depth of the research project could be understood. However, it is inadequate to fully comprehend the "everyday" realities of the lives of Caribbean women and, in particular, working-class women. Section 2 focuses on the process of data collection which was crucial in accessing valid information that not only acknowledged the importance of this innovative process, but made sure that the women's voices were retained.

Notes

1. The terms post-colonial state, peripheral state and neo- colonial state are used interchangeably since all three concepts explain the underlying structural relationships present in these societies after the attainment of constitutional independence.
2. Lydia Pulsipher. "He won't let she stretch she foot: Gender Relations in Traditional West Indian Houseyards." (eds.), Cindi Katz and Janice Monk Full Circles: *Geographies of Women over the Life Course.* London & New York: Routledge, 1993:108.
3. See Mohammed and Shepherd (1988); Green (1992); Reddock (1991); Bush (1990); Beckles(1989); Morrissey (1989); Senior (1991); Momsen (1993); Brereton (1988).
4. Bridget Brereton. "General Problems and Issues in Studying the History of Women." (eds.) Patricia Mohammed and Catherine Shepherd, *Gender in Caribbean Development.*:Mona, Jamaica; St. Augustine, Trinidad and Tobago; Cave Hill, Barbados: The University of the West Indies Women and Development Project, 1988:123.
5. Ibid.:123-124.
6. Ibid.:127.
7. Ibid.
8. Ibid.:128.
9. Ibid.:130.
10. Ibid.:131.
11. Ibid.:134.
12. Ibid.:135.
13. Ibid.
14. Rosina Wiltshire-Brodber. "Gender, Race and Class in the Caribbean." (eds.) Patricia Mohammed and Catherine Shepherd, *Gender in Caribbean Development.* Mona, Jamaica; St. Augustine, Trinidad and Tobago; Cave Hill, Barbados: The University Of The West Indies Women and Development Project, 1988:147.
15. See V. Vargas. "The Women's Movement in Peru." (eds.) Sarah A. Radcliffe and Sally Westwood, Viva: *Women and Popular Protest in Latin America.*:Routledge & Kegan Paul, 1993

(1990):1.

16. Ibid.: 1-2.
17. See Ben Fine. *Women's Employment and Capitalist Family*. London: Routledge & Kegan Paul, 1992: 22.
18. Ibid.
19. Walby cited in Ben Fine, 23-24.
20. Ibid.:23-24; see also S. Rowbotham (1972).
21. Ibid.:23-24.
22. Ibid.
23. Ibid.
24. Ibid.:24.
25. V. Vargas (1993):1.
26. Ibid.:1-2.
27. Marietta Morrissey. *Slave Women in the New World: Gender Stratification in the Caribbean*.: University Press of Kansas, 1989: 1X.
28. Ibid.
29. Ibid.:X-XI.
30. Ibid.
31. Cecilia Green. "Reclaiming Women's Lives." *Gender and Re\Production in West Indian Slaves Societies, Part 1: Against the Current:* September/October, 1992: 31.
32. Orlando Patterson. "Persistence, Continuity, and Change in the Jamaican Working-Class Family." *Journal of Family History,* 7:1982:135-161.
33. Patterson quoted by Green, C., op cit., pp. 31-32.
34. Patterson quoted by Green, C., op cit., p.32.
35. Ibid.
36. Green, op cit., p. 32.
37. Ibid.
38. Ibid.
39. Ibid.:32-33.
40. Ibid.:33-35.
41. Beckles (1991) quoted by Cecilia Greene, p. 34.
42. Green, op cit., p.33-35.
43. Ibid.: 35; see also Barbara Bush (1982, 1990).
44. J. Tucker 1990:219.
45. Ibid.: 223.
46. Ibid.
47. Ibid.
48. Ibid.:199.
49. Ibid.
50. Michael Davis. "Colonial Discourses, Representation and the Construction of Otherness: Case Studies from Papua,": Mangilao, Guam: (ed.) Donald H. Rubinstein, *Pacific History Papers from*

the 8th Pacific History Association Conference, (University of Guam Press & Micronesian Area research Center, 1992):49.

51. Green, Cecilia. (1992):32.
52. Rhoda Reddock. "New Developments in Research on Women: The Commonwealth Caribbean Experience." *Women Studies International: Nairobi and Beyond*, New York: The Feminist Press, 1991:159.
53. See Clarke (1986); Durant-Gonsalvez (1976) Powell (1989); Odi-Ali (1986).
54. See Davies (1987); Rogers (1980); Senior (1991) Ford-Smith (1991) and others.
55. See Wireinga (1988); Miles (1988); Bulbeck (1988); Mohanthy (1991).

SECTION 2:
THE CARIBBEAN STATE,
HEALTH CARE AND
WOMEN

Section 1 provided the theoretical framework in which the lives of Caribbean women, would be considered. Section 2 builds on this framework, providing a comprehensive context in which to examine the women's history, political influence, socio-economic status and specifically their health status.

Chapter 4, looks at the methodology used and the rationale behind the study design. Chapter 5, which presents a historical overview of women in the Caribbean, specifically looks at their socio-economic and health status from the first European discovery of the Caribbean, through slavery, apprenticeship, emancipation, colonialism, pre-independence and independence. The next two chapters paint a global picture of the states under study. The analysis concentrates on the political, socio-economic and health environments during the period of 1979 to 1983, although in some cases a historical overview is necessary to put the assessment in perspective. Chapter 6 is dedicated to a review of Barbados, while Chapter 7 presents a discussion of the situation in Grenada. For consistency in argument and comparison, both chapters are developed using a similar structure and are presented as follows:

1. A brief overview of the political climate prior to 1979 followed by a more detailed look at the political ideologies and activities between 1979 to 1983.

2. An account of the prevailing economic situation which highlights key statistics and problems and looks at key economic policy development.

3. An assessment of women's status and their relationship with the state, including an examination of some of the legislation implemented during the period.

4. An examination of how these two ideologically different states implemented the Primary Health Care (PHC) Model in accordance with the Alma Ata Declaration of 1978. Under this umbrella, certain aspects of their health care systems are examined: the health infrastructure; the health budget and allocation of capital resources; the health policy and administration, specifically the model of PHC developed.

An assessment of the health care policies and delivery systems in the two states begins in Chapter 8 which provides a critique of the system from a professional viewpoint. The assessment continues in Chapter 9 which presents the viewpoint of working class women and includes a detailed profile of this selected group of health care consumers.

CHAPTER 4

EMPIRICAL RESEARCH METHODOLOGY

Chapter 4 explains the choice of research areas and time period. It outlines the methodology used to investigate the health care policy and service development in Barbados and Grenada and its impact on women, particularly working class women.

SELECTION OF RESEARCH AREAS

Barbados is unique in the Caribbean in that it had a long unbroken British colonial rule (1625-1966) and was the only island which had a resident white planter class. It was also one of the few islands to be inhabited only by Black slaves and White planters, without traces of a resident indigenous population or later, as was true for other islands, other indentured peoples. This situation created a rigid class and racial structure comprised of the economically advantaged White minority plantocracy at the top, and the black masses, the majority of whom were plantation labourers, at the bottom.

Grenada, on the other hand, was ruled by both the British and the French. The island has a violent history, with internal class and race conflicts and popular rebellions dating back as far as 1650. Unlike Barbados, but like many other Caribbean islands (such as St. Lucia, St. Vincent and Dominica), the Black population was predominantly based in the rural areas and owned their own land on which they cultivated cash-crops and food for the family. This arrangement undergirded the social and cultural development of the Grenadian people and influenced the way in which conflicts that threatened their ownership were settled.

Although both states experienced colonial rule and are considered "small nations," they differ drastically with respect to their political ideology and economic status. Barbados, a liberal democratic state, is considered one of the More Developed Countries (MDCs)[1] in the Caribbean and ranks high in terms of education, health and other social services compared to other countries in the entire region; while Grenada, a repressive state prior to the focal period of the study, is considered a Lesser Developed Country (LDC).[2] *(Table 4.1 summarizes key demographic and health statistics for Barbados and Grenada).* Political and economic differences have influenced the development of health care systems in the two countries, a fact that made the two states attractive for this study as contrasting models.

The selection of Barbados and Grenada also stemmed from a number of personal and professional interests. I was a resident familiar with Barbados, where I resided from 1980 to 1989. From 1980-1983, under the tenure of the Barbados Labour Party Government (BLP) I served as a public service employee. In 1983, upon leaving government service, I joined the Women and Development Unit (WAND) of the University of the West Indies. I had close contacts with a number of individuals who were part of the Grenada Government from 1979 to 1983 and subsequently worked in Grenada as a WAND Program Officer, from 1983-87. During my work experience in Grenada, I became interested in whether women were perceived differently in a revolutionary state versus other post-colonial states in the English-speaking Caribbean, specifically Barbados. My professional and scholarly interest, which finally formed the basis for my research, was to examine how these two ideologically and structurally different States: Barbados and Grenada, approached health policy development, and to determine how those policies were beneficial or detrimental to the health and perceived well-being of the

Table 4.1
Barbados and Grenada: Selected Demographic and Health Statistics, 1979–1983 and 1984–1993

STATISTICS	BARBADOS	GRENADA
Location	Most easterly of Caribbean Islands	Most southerly of the Windward Islands
Size (area)	166 square miles (21 miles long by 14 miles wide); mostly flat, highest point is 1,105 feet[3]	120 square miles (21 miles long by 12 miles wide); 133 square miles (including dependencies); highest peak is approx. 2,756 feet above sea level[4]
Capital City	Bridgetown	St. George's
Language	English	English; Patois (local)

Statistic	BARBADOS 1979–1983	BARBADOS 1984–1993	GRENADA 1979–1983	GRENADA 1984–1993
Population:				
Total	253,000	254,300	89,088	94,746
Female	132,000	132,859	46,145	48,169
Male	121,000	122,561	42,943	46,577
Ethnic Groups (%):				
Black	87.9	87.9	80.0	82.0
Mixed			10.0	
East Indian	0.8	0.8	3.0	
Other	11.3	11.3	7.0	18.0*
Life Expectancy at Birth:				
Total Population	70.0	-	65.5	69
Women	72.3	75.2		72
Men	67.2	70.2		66
Infant Mortality Rate (per 1000 live births)	24.5	17.7	21.2	25.05

*includes Mixed, East Indian Nationals, Whites and other groups.

Sources: (1) Jules, Didacus (1992); (2) UNICEF Caribbean Area Office, "Draft Situational Analysis of Children and Women in Grenada"; (3) Annual Reports of the Chief Medical Officer of Health, 1984, 1989, 1991; (4) Porter, Rosemary (1986); (5) Notes on Population and Development in Grenada, Planning Unit of Grenada.

women. My engagement with both Barbados and Grenada gave me the unique opportunity to examine them from both an "insider" and "outsider" position. This book grew out of insights and by using a combination of historical and empirical material.

RESEARCH PROCEDURE

In December, 1991, I was awarded the Young Canadian Researcher Award (YCRA) from IDRC (International Development Research Council). I became affiliated with the University of the West Indies Campus in Barbados with Dr. Hilary Beckles, a historian, as my field supervisor. Barbados became my main base, giving me ready access to various regional and international bodies.

To begin the process of inquiry, in May 1992, introductory letters were sent to the Director of the Bureau of Women's Affairs at the Ministry of Community Development and Culture in Barbados and the Minister for Tourism, Civil Aviation and Women's Affairs in Grenada. These persons were informed of my research and their support was solicited in gaining access to key organizations and agencies. Partial lists of potential interviewees were sent, and this allowed the Barbadian Ministry to contact a number of potential government and non-governmental personnel on my behalf and to set-up a tentative appointment schedule prior to my arrival in Barbados at the end of August 1992. Permission to interview women who used the state health facilities was requested from the Chief Medical Officer of Health, the Medical Officers of Health of the assigned sites and the women themselves.

In Barbados, I conducted interviews with key local health care providers, representatives of women's organizations, trade unions, and regional and international bodies working in the area of health and related fields from a regional perspective (including UNICEF, the Pan-American Health Organization (PAHO), and the Caribbean Development Bank (CDB)). In Barbados, officials of the Barbados Labour Party were seen, as well as the incumbent Democratic Labour Party Government. In Grenada, I spoke with members of both current and former members of the People's Revolutionary Government. Clearance was obtained for visits to the Polyclinics in Barbados and Grenada to interview their staff and clients.

METHODOLOGY AND METHODOLOGICAL ISSUES

The study adopts a multi-level method approach. It assesses "women's lives during and after slavery, as well as women's struggles against human oppression"[5] in order to examine the development and impact of state health policy on women. The method is in essence sociological, but possesses several socio-historical characteristics which contribute to its uniqueness; it integrates a historical approach (analysis of official documents and records, reading of texts, articles, etc.), standard sociological structured interviews, and anthropological, unstructured in-depth interviewing techniques in the achievement of responsible research.[6]

This interdisciplinary approach facilitated a comprehensive and holistic understanding of women's concrete situation in the countries under study. It began by examining the historical data, followed by governing current perceptions about the health care system, its policies and services, and then looked at the underlying medical and political assumptions that guided these states' health policies. To ensure that the "voices" of women were not muted by the intrusion of traditional mainstream methodological research tools and expectations, open-ended, semi-structured interviews were used with the group of women because they more easily allow outsiders to "explore peoples' views of reality and allow the research to generate theory."[7] Barbadian and Grenadian women "expert-informants" were central to the research process, which ultimately sought to understand their perspectives on primary health care services. An unusual dimension of the study is that people were asked to reflect on aspects of health care policy implemented and services delivered a decade before and to compare those with the current health policies and services. As such, one stipulation made for selection of these interviewees was that the candidates had to be at least over the age of twenty. Utilitzing the unique interdisciplinary method described above, the intensive field study carried out in

Barbados and Grenada from September 1992 to February 1993 proved its ability to show the impact of the period 1979 to 1983 on the lives of Black working-class women, interestingly far beyond just providing insights into the health picture alone.

Debate

The choice in methodology, which places emphasis on "the individuals under study rather than on the research itself," has been influenced by Bolles.[8] Further, as noted by Etter-Lewis, "when applied to women of color, it assumes added significance as a powerful instrument for the rediscovery of womanhood so often overlooked and/or neglected in history and literature alike."[9] To engage in information-gathering that is not superficial, but which aspires to a robust approximation of "truth," the researcher must be fully knowledgeable about "the historical, cultural, economic and political dynamics of the society under examination,"[10] and purposefully unveil the gender dynamics too. According to Harley, one way of ensuring that the voices of African women from the continent and African women from the Diaspora are heard is for researchers and development analysts to adopt an "insider" perspective.[11] This research approach dictates that the researcher study the experiences and perspectives of the group being analyzed based on the group's reality rather than on the researcher's reality when the two are distinct.[12] This is particularly true for working-class women who often have their reality interpreted for them by researchers.

Sources

The primary sources of data came from the interviews with the working class Barbadian and Grenadian women and with the health providers, administrators and policy makers, as well as from several original documents (laws and legislation, government publications, official reports). Other sources of data included state Development Plans; health services development plans; Central Bank Reports; chief medical officers' Annual Reports; budget speeches; documents of the Barbados Association of Medical Practitioners (BAMP); reports from regional and international agencies based in Barbados and the Grenadian papers, now housed at Marryshow House, School of Continuing Studies, University of the West Indies.

Interviews

Barbados: Interviews were conducted during office hours in the month of September with representatives from the Ministry of Health (including the Minister and ex-Minister of Health), the Women's Bureau and other Women Organizations, BAMP hospital and polyclinic staff, UWI Medical School faculty, regional and international organizations, and trade unions.

In Barbados, two polyclinics (one large urban based clinic and one smaller rural based one) were recommended as suitable sites for examination by the Medical Officer of Health since their users were representative of the female Barbadian population. At each clinic, prepatory time was dedicated to talking with staff, observing how the clinic functioned, and preparing a schedule for interviewing the polyclinic-users. Staff suggested interviewing on the days in which several clinics operated simultaneously to facilitate a varied sample in terms of age and presenting medical problems. Working-class women between the ages of 30-55 were selected from case files (by the senior nurse) or were asked (by me or by the nursing personnel) if they would like to take part in the study. Generally they were willing. Similarly, to gain the perspective of women who used private clinics, the cooperation of two private practitioners was obtained to find women within a similar age group who would be willing to participate in the study. (The same age criterion was used as a way of maintaining consistency with the polyclinic women). The private clinic interviews were more difficult to arrange and were not completed until November, 1992.

Grenada: During the month of October 1992 interviews were conducted with personnel from the Ministry of Health, Women's Bureau, School of Continuing Education (University of the West Indies), non-governmental organizations (NGOs); and former members of the National Women's Organization (NWO), the PRG administration and women supporters who worked in the PRG. Two members of the staff volunteered assistance and contacted personnel by telephone. A guarantee of anomynity wasa condition insisted upon by most of the interviewees. Quite a number of the professionals had to be interviewed outside of working hours or at weekends to maintain the level of confidentiality.

In order to get a broad cross section of views from Grenadian working class women, the final sites selected consisted of three rural health stations including one in Carriacou (a separate island which with Grenada and Petite Martinique forms the country of Grenada), and one urban health centre. Grenada, unlike Barbados, consists of a large rural-based population. It took several hours by car to reach rural health stations, and it was often necessary to make more than one trip to complete an interview. Women from both Grenada and Carriacou who used private health care services instead of public care were also interviewed. In order to carry out interviews in Carriacou, I traveled for about three hours one way by ferry. The same methods used for selecting and interviewing the women who used state owned polyclinics and private doctors' clinics in Barbados were utilized in Grenada.

Interviews with the professional group entailed a more structured approach. Questions solicited respondents' perceptions of the government's declared health care policy, particularly with regard to women's health as a key area of focus. In addition some supplementary questions were prepared for key individuals in the health field and at the Bureau of Women's Affairs. The Barbadian and Grenadian working class women interviewed were asked to critique the health care system of their respective countries and to comment on the states' sensitivity to their health care needs, as (working class) women.

Description of Sample

A total of one hundred[13] interviews were conducted with Barbadian and Grenadian women and men of various political views and socio-economic backgrounds. The sample represented a wide cross-section of opinions and views of the populations (middle class and working class) in Barbados and Grenada. All interviews were taped and were transcribed over a four month period. Forty professionals were interviewed, twenty-five (62.5%) of whom were women. In-depth interviews were conducted with a total of sixty working class women, twenty-seven (45%)

Barbadian and thirty-three (55%) Grenadians. Grenada, unlike Barbados, has a large rural population and therefore, to include representation from both rural and urban areas, more women from Grenada than Barbados were interviewed.

Data Analysis

A stronger emphasis was placed on qualitative methods rather than on quantitative methods. Qualitative findings were supported by quantitative data. Themes which emerged from the questions posed to the women and professionals were used to group the responses into categories. All categories therefore emerged inductively from the data instead of being pre-set.[14]

RESEARCH CHALLENGES

Four main challenges were experienced during the data collection process. The first was the unavailability of some primary documents. This problem was most prominent in Grenada where several PRG government documents had either been removed by the US State Department during the invasion in 1983 or had been destroyed. In addition, the photocopies of some of the documents returned to Grenada by the US after the invasion were in such poor condition they proved useless to the study. Some supplementary information on Grenada was found at regional and international agencies located in Barbados.

Second, government documents, especially in developing societies, are known to be unreliable in that they often reflect the class and patriarchal perspectives and biases of the dominant strata. Accordingly, most of the statistical data necessary to assess the health status of women in the region is not disaggregated.[15] For example, mortality data is not stratified by gender and age, and official documents often fail "to include the female presence other than in passing."[16]

Despite the paucity of quantitative data, I believe the study's results did not suffer. The limitations were overcome by utilizing qualitative data as the main source and quantitative data as a supplementary source (rather than vice versa). In addition, the methodology provided the context for the quantitative and qualitative data acquired within the historical, political and socio-economic development of the two states, and this "multi-level approach" contributed to a more holistic understanding of the issues facing working class Barbadian and Grenadian women.

Third, since the study was situated in the 1979 to 1983 period, the conclusions drawn from qualitative data depended on the ability of interviewees to accurately remember the events that occurred in their states. This "accurate memory" concept was particularly sensitive for Grenadians. They were being asked to recall a traumatic historical period in their lives and their recall may, at times, have been skewed. This potential problem was tempered by using the multi-level approach, referred to earlier, and through the range of people interviewed. Professionals from all levels of the administrative and power hierarchy, government and non-government personnel and working class women from the city as well as rural areas were interviewed, and in the case of Grenada, proportionately more Grenadian working class women were interviewed than Barbadian working class women. Thus a claim made by at least two persons from the same or different groupings (stronger if the latter) can be considered more or less reliable.

Fourth, since the research is an original, it required the collection of new data and information. Few studies have been done that look at gender in relation to the state and health care policy and service delivery. I, therefore, had to find creative but methodologically rigourous ways of obtaining information relevant to the study, which proved to be challenging at times.

Notes

1.   The MDCs include: Trinidad & Tobago, Jamaica, Barbados, Guyana, Belize and Bahamas See LeRoy Taylor, (1990).

2.   The LDCs include: St Lucia, Dominica, St. Christopher-Nevis (St. Kitts), St. Vincent & the Grenadines, Antigua & Barbuda, Monsterrat and Grenada. See Taylor, LeRoy, 1990.

3.   see Annual Report of Chief Medical Officer of Health, Ministry of Health, Barbados, 1984.

4.   UNICEF, Caribbean Area Office, "Draft Situation Analysis of Children and Women in Grenada," Barbados 1991

5.   Rosalyn Terborg-Penn (ed). "African Feminism: A Theoretical Approach to the History of Women in the African Diaspora" in

Women in Africa and the African Diaspora, Howard University Press. 1987:50.

6. See Bolles, (1987).
7. Janet Finch "Feminist Research and Social Policy", (eds.) Mavis Maclean & Dulcie Graves, *Women Isues in Social Policy,* London & NY: Routledge, 1991:18.
8. See Bolles, (1987); (1993).
9. Gwendolyn Etter-Lewis "Black Women's Life Stories: Reclaiming Self in Narrative Texts." (eds.) Sherna Berger Gluck and Daphne Patai, *Women's Words: The Feminist Practice of Oral History*, New York and London: Routledge and Kegan Paul, 1991:43; *see* also Patricia Hill-Collins (1991).
10. Harley, Sharon "Research Priorities for the Study of Women in Africa and the Diaspora.(eds.). Gwendolyn Terberg-Penn ; Sharon Harley; Andrea Benton Rushing, *Women in Africa and the African Diaspora,* Howard University Press, 1987:211.
11. Harley, Sharon, "Research Priorities for the study of Women in Africa and the Diaspora(eds.) Rosalyn Terberg-Penn et al *Women in Africa and the Diaspora,* Howard University Press, 1987: 211; *see* also Barbara Omolade (1990).
12. Sharon Harley (1987).
13. This number is statistically significant; sample sizes equal to or greater than 30 are considered large.
14. See Buvinic et al (1979).
15. see Gloria Beckles (1992):13.
16. Rosalyn Terborg-Penn; Sharon Harley; Andrea Benton Rushing, eds (1987):43.

CHAPTER 5

HISTORICAL OVERVIEW OF WOMEN'S HEALTH IN THE CARIBBEAN

This chapter provides a historical overview of the socio-economic development of the English-speaking Caribbean region and the growth of health care policy in regard to women. *(See Appendix 1 for Map of the Caribbean Region)* It also provides a platform from which to examine more recent developments in the Caribbean, particularly in Barbados and Grenada, with respect to women's roles and status, state health policy and service delivery and the state's willingness/ability to meet the health care needs of women. The assessment shows that the experiences of exploitation and underdevelopment over centuries has had far-reaching effects for the societies which emerged and still impact on the lives of women today.

Several historical studies documented the inhuman conditions slaves were forced to endure during their transportation to the Caribbean where they were forcibly set to work on sugar plantations. The health of Caribbean people was compromised from the beginning; and of the estimated "ten million Africans transported.... an average of 13 to 33 percent died"[1] as a result of the poor and callous conditions, beatings, lack of insufficient care and suicides. The Caribbean region can, therefore, be considered to be founded on a racist ideology and practice, one which was used to rationalize slavery and to institutionalize a mercantilist-based capitalist society. These two systems collectively succeeded in economically exploiting, physically harming and emotionally abusing not only slaves and working peoples but also indigenous peoples. Based on the WHO definition of health and the view that health constitutes the total well-being of an individual, it can be argued that the Caribbean society started off with men and women who were deprived of positive health influences and were as a result physically and psychologically unwell.

The following is an examination of the health conditions of Caribbean peoples, particularly those of women, from Columbus' arrival in the Caribbean, through the periods of slavery, apprenticeship, emancipation, colonialism, pre-independence and independence.

PRE-SLAVERY (1492 to 1643)

Christopher Columbus (a Spaniard) arrived in the Caribbean Islands, opening up new virgin territory to be exploited by Europeans. Spain became the forerunner in the enslavement of the native peoples who were "subjected to gross indignities which were alien to their nature." [2] The enslavement of the Native people was not instant, but entailed a long and protracted struggle between the invaders and the invaded. Some resisted enslavement by using such methods as infanticide and suicide or seeking refuge in the hills; the majority, however, died as a result of overwork in the gold mines and susceptibility to the variety of diseases brought by the Europeans. For the Native peoples, this era marked their "gradual depletion which was soon to end in their almost complete extinction from the West Indies." [3]

With the decimation of the Native inhabitants, the Europeans turned to an exported labour force. Initially, the recruitment of labour was based on some of the surviving Amerindians (as they were referred to), Europeans who were fleeing religious and political persecution in their homelands, Africans and Asians. The large scale production envisaged, however, required a much larger and cheaper source of labour. The slave trade provided such a solution; Africans were transported from the continent to the Caribbean in extraordinary and inhuman conditions, forming the backbone of the Caribbean economy for a period lasting over two hundred years.

SLAVERY (1644 to 1833)

The 'slave' period was critical in establishing the class, race and gender discriminations that would later on become embedded in the psyche of Caribbean people and remain difficult to change. The society "was stratified into white, brown and black which corresponded to the social and economic structure."[4] This deep seated racism had a negative impact on the lives of the Black population. The general health, well being and

> longevity of African West Indian slaves were related both directly and indirectly to their living conditions and the medical services they received ....What existed was a vicious circle of disease and racism whereby the debility of blacks was often misconstrued by planters and doctors as racial characteristics of laziness and shamming illness.[5]

The slave trade and slavery were justified by the oppressors by erecting a negative stereotype of the Caribbean African man and woman. Black slaves were portrayed as inferior to their White masters; this set in motion the institutionalization of racial prejudice, discrimination and oppression, and centuries of colonialization which have affected the mental well being and self-esteem of many of the region's peoples.

Recent research in Canada has indicated that "[r]acism has far reaching health consequences"[6] and as such health and mental health systems need to be developed in order to "enable people to heal from racial abuse."[7] In 1992 at the Annual General Meeting of the Ontario Public Health Association (OPHA), the Working Group on Economic and Social Justice put forward a resolution on anti-racism in health; the resolution was unanimously passed by the OPHA membership and a number of initiatives are now (1993) being considered as the "awareness of racism as a health issue ... [with] far reaching health consequences"[8] increases. This new perspective on the racism-health relationship makes it necessary for health professionals, in general, to become more sensitive to the health concerns of ethnocultural groups. In the case of Caribbean peoples and particularly the women, this is important, and

> requires an understanding of the social relations underlying slavery since these relations of power and inequality continue to exist despite the strides made.[9]

Health care services being directed at Black women and women of colour must recognize and be sensitive to those negative aspects of their historical past which perpetuated self-hatred and low-self esteem, and resulted in internalized racism and to their disempowerment.[10]

As may be expected, a centralized health policy did not exist during slavery. Slaves were the property of their owners and were seen, first and foremost, as commodities. For example, sick slaves were attended to at their master's convenience. Slaves who complained of being ill were ignored and denied food, an action which perpetuated their conditions and impaired their capacity to work. To compensate for this deficiency, the slaves relied heavily on their traditional healing methods (as did non-slave poor and working class groups). Afro-Caribbean medicine played an important role not just for medical practices, but was also used, in combination with religion and folk culture, as a survival strategy. These forms of worship and care, although viewed as "primitive" by the planters and the church, were practiced widely and the cultures they represented survived because of the diverse modes of transmission used. Information was passed through the household, multi-household (extended family), the ethnic church, the folk clinic and voluntary organizations, and women played a key role in passing knowledge through their daughters, with whom they shared close relationships.[10] Records show that Black nurses often had to combine their supervisory and professional roles with menial duties in order to provide continuous care to the injured and sick slaves in plantation hospitals (this was necessary because of the infrequent visits made by white doctors and overseers).[11] Unfortunately, there were no records of the health care provided by women to their sick family members and friends; however, it may be assumed that, since slaves were not admitted to hospital until they were almost dead, the majority of care was delivered outside of the hospital setting.

African men and women, although their dietary allowances were unequal, were treated as equal producers. On many estates, during hard times, both male and female slaves were made to do an excess of manual work such as hoeing and weeding. During these periods, women were also responsible for finding food for themselves and their families; many resorted to theft as a means of survival. On plantations in Barbados women rarely survived beyond 50 to 55 years, and when they did they were so worn out that they were confined to providing child care services. Beckles noted that, despite legislation, not all of these older women were allowed to stay on the plantations and many of them were forced to survive as best as they could on their own.[12] Slaves who were unable to produce were either sold for a nominal fee as domestic help to poor whites, or even to "free Blacks."[13]

Black women who worked as unskilled labourers on the sugar plantations experienced both physical and psychological trauma during slavery. They suffered through excessive labour (They were expected to do heavy manual work as well as to work night shifts in the boiling house.[14]), punishment, malnutrition, vulnerability to disease, high mortality and fear of abandonment when they were no longer able to work. "Sexual exploitation and violence were inescapable features of the black woman's condition."[16] They were victimized because of their sex and many, raped by the ship's crews, had arrived in the Caribbean already pregnant.

Sheridan noted that some plantation owners were unsympathetic to the toll this suffering took on women emotionally, physically and especially reproductively. In fact, plantation owners disapproved of pregnancy; not only did it remove the woman from the labour force, but it was more expensive to financially support a mother and child. Importation of new slaves proved much cheaper than the rearing of children who, in any case, were not productive before the age of five years. Pregnant women were nevertheless made to work in the field during the last month of pregnancy and this, in combination with frequent whippings and malnutrition, contributed to the high rates of miscarriages. Even those who miscarried were expected to return to work almost immediately. As a result of these cruel and unjust conditions, resistance became a central part of the everyday life of the Black women. Rather than have their children enslaved and suffer the same injustices, many women underwent crude abortions or committed infanticide.[15] These conditions no doubt affected their physical, emotional and mental health, and consequently their ability to lead "healthy" lives.

APPRENTICESHIP (1834 to 1838)

In 1833, through the Imperial Act of Parliament, provision was made "that children under six years of age should be free but that all other slaves should serve a period of apprenticeship."[16] Apprenticeship was instituted at the end of the period of slavery in all British Commonwealth colonies (and in other legislative colonies) as a gradual process towards emancipation,[17] and was to have lasted until 1840. This transition period (a compromise between the British Government and the planter class) was deemed necessary to give the slaves time to adjust to their new status of freedom[18], to ensure that the Caribbean was safe for the continued operation and long term survival of the sugar plantations, and to implement the emancipation legislation. The "apprentice" field workers were required to work for six years and domestic slaves for a period of four years before emancipation. During this period, the newly emancipated men and women were required to work, for free, for three-fourths of the week (40 1/2 hours) and were paid only for the remaining fourth. From these meager wages, they were supposed to save enough money to buy their freedom; this could be done at anytime before the end of their apprenticeship period.

The British government, aware of the treatment of the slaves during slavery, passed laws that were supposed to protect the apprentices. For example, they limited the power of the owners to punish, and prohibited flogging and the working of apprentices on Sundays. Instead plantation owners were required to provide religious instruction, "food, clothing, lodging, medicine and medical attendance for the apprentice or, in lieu of food, adequate provision ground and time in which to cultivate them."[19] In exchange, the apprentice had to "live up to the contract, work honestly, and refrain from insolence and insubordination."[20]

However, despite the supposedly protective measures, little changed. Most of the new laws represented a double standard and were not actively enforced; some of the people responsible for administering the legislation were not only sympathetic to the planters but were often slave owners themselves![21] Labourers who were late for work lost half a day's wage, and those absent for two or more days within a week, or accused of bad work and/or laziness were punished by a magistrate. Even the labour of children was exploited and parents who tried to prevent their children from working were fined. This outright disregard for the terms of emancipation was a show of power by the planter class, and was used as a delaying tactic to extend the apprenticeship period and maximize the exploitation of the ex-slaves before their freedom.

Thus, despite the claim that slavery was officially abolished, the apprenticeship period in effect proved to be a time of "modified slavery."[22] The socio-economic and health conditions of the Afro-Caribbean people had not improved. During slavery, the owners had a responsibility to provide at least minimal care, food and protection; now, the ex-slaves/apprentices were expected to support themselves on the meagre wages they received for their labour. Housing was still owned and controlled by the planters and subject to arbitrary rentals. For example, instead of charging the labourers a fixed rent, the owners charged each occupant of the house.[23] The health conditions of the ex-slaves also deteriorated as rudimentary medical services, first-aid, and medication formerly provided by the plantation owners were now no longer available. The region continued to be plagued with epidemics and suffered several outbreaks of cholera in the 1850s. In Barbados in 1854, 20,000 people (nearly all Black or Coloured[24]) died; in Jamaica, the cholera epidemic of 1850 was estimated to have killed between 25,000 to 30,000 people and was tragically followed by an outbreak of smallpox and then by another bout of cholera.[25] The ex-slaves, therefore, continued to live and work under severe, "unhealthy" conditions.

FULL EMANCIPATION (1838 to 1900)

The Emancipation Act passed on August 1, 1834, finally became a reality on June 2, 1838. The Caribbean society by that time had a rigid class, race and gender hierarchy in place. In the position of power was a small group of White men who controlled the economic and political state mechanisms. The group included officials, plantation owners, merchants and professional men, attorneys, overseers, bookkeepers and master craftsmen. The second group consisted of a large number of Coloureds whose rights as citizens were limited; although they were allowed to own property, carry arms, and to give evidence in a court of law, they were denied the right to vote or to contest an election. At the bottom of the pyramid were the approximately 750,000 ex-slaves[26], Blacks who had very few rights at all. They were, for example, still denied the use of the segregated city hospitals and therefore continued to rely on the indigenous forms of medical care which had thrived during slavery, and on the women as critical paid and unpaid care providers.

The freed slaves, however, now had three choices: to continue working on the plantations, to work for themselves, or to leave the region. Those who chose to continue working for plantation owners could now sell their labour to whichever plantation paid the best wages, and this practice resulted in increased labour cost and consequently a decline in the profits realized from the sugar industry. Those who chose to work for themselves turned to small scale farming. Prior to emancipation, this was done only by run-away slaves, such as the Maroons and independent Blacks who squatted on Crown lands. Later, to escape the poor working conditions experienced under the hands of plantation owners, more and more ex-slaves turned to small-scale farming as a means of survival. Small farms subsequently began to thrive and the resulting new peasantry which developed struggled to co-exist within the much larger social system that continued to be dominated by the plantation owners. The obvious growth and potential of the small farmers threatened the status quo, raising the plantation owners' concerns as they saw a depletion in their cheap labour supply. Thus, in order to survive, the plantation owners collaborated with the State machinery, and military and paramilitary troops were used to destroy crops which were not grown on the plantations, and to seize animals that were raised without their permission. This was in direct contrast to policies which were encouraged and adopted in the non-plantation or "settler" colonies in North America (including Canada), Australia and New Zealand where families were encouraged and provided with assistance to expand and settle.[27]

Many Black Caribbean people migrated to Panama (to work on the Canal), Costa Rica, Cuba, Britain and the USA in search of a better life, and, consequently, the labour supply shrunk drastically. Financial and labour constraints limited the planters' capacity to cover operational costs and forced them from 1838 to 1924 to import a cheaper labour pool, indentured labourers mainly from India[28], and to rely more on female labour. During the period 1891 to 1921, when young men were emigrating, the total female labour force in Barbados climbed from 57% to 61%; most were employed in the agricultural sector, although a large number also worked as domestics, milliners and seamstresses, petty traders and shopkeepers.[29] Already overworked, the increased responsibility of being sole economic provider no doubt increased the stress of these women.

PRE-INDEPENDENCE ERA (1900 to 1960)

1900 to 1940

The entire state apparatus was "arrayed against the emancipated slaves"[30] and their efforts to establish a 'free' life were blocked at all angles. Paradoxically, this continued domination of the "free-slaves" increased their determination for freedom. As a direct consequence, revolts and a series of rebellions began to occur throughout the English-speaking Caribbean region between 1934 to 1939. The British government responded by appointing a Royal Commission of Inquiry, the Moyne Commission, to investigate the causes for the disturbances. Perhaps without these struggles, the inhuman conditions which the working peoples endured and survived would not have been documented, and action may not have been taken when it was, to redress the situation.

The Moyne Report[31] characterized the health situation

among the Black population, in most territories, as one of high infant and maternal mortality. Many of the prevalent communicable diseases resulted from the poor living conditions and lack of public facilities including adequate water supplies and sanitation services. According to the Report, the housing conditions in both urban and rural areas were "unfit for human occupation"; the situation was worse in the densely populated urban centres where makeshift dwellings, overcrowding, imperfect ventilation and lack of sanitary facilities contributed to the spread of tuberculosis, several intestinal and respiratory diseases and numerous sexually transmitted diseases. The tradition of poor housing was a left-over from slavery when plantation owners tried to reduce the cost of housing the slaves. Emancipation encouraged the development of large villages and towns, and migration to these areas led to large scale overcrowding in the urban areas. The situation was further exacerbated by the absence of a coherent housing policy and state welfare program. The rudimentary welfare services that existed were organized to a large extent by the churches and voluntary organizations.

Although the Report highlighted the severity of the population's existence, disappointingly, it was more descriptive than analytical. The document is the only one of its kind that provided a detailed account of the poverty, ill-health and structural conditions under which the Caribbean poor lived in the 1930s. The recommendations, however, were merely palliative since the Report "consistently failed to address the root causes of the peoples' distress....it was neither revolutionary nor radical"[32] and neglected to deal with the vicious socio-economic cycle which the working class was trapped.

The economic situation and social conditions of the working class did not improve under the colonial state. The region suffered from high unemployment and there was a large population of poorly paid workers. This impoverished economic situation manifested itself in substandard housing, inadequate public health measures, poor nutrition, and poor health-conditions which impacted on the population's productivity and that of the region as a whole. Wages in 1938 (although much higher than those between 1923 to 33) remained extremely low, with the most common per day wage for an unskilled sugar worker being 28 cents in St. Vincent, 23-26 cents in St. Kitts-Nevis, 30-48 cents in Grenada, 35 cents in Trinidad and 48-60 cents in Jamaica.[33] Throughout the region, both government and private employers adopted a policy of "rotational" employment. For example, a worker would be given work for a fortnight and then discharged to make room for someone else. Although each country had a different method of combating the problem, the instability made it hard to earn a decent wage; this, in conjunction with the high cost of locally grown food, made it impossible for people to eat a nutritious diet. The high cost of food is attributable to the imbalance in land available for locally used food versus crops grown for export and the consequent dependency on importation as a means of providing the population with basic foods. In Trinidad, for instance, a labourer was dependent "on external sources for 80 percent of his food"[34]; and in Barbados, the local diet consisted of imported rice and cornmeal.

Although the entire population suffered, there was systematic gender discrimination. Women were not only paid less than the men for the same work, but were also given less rations and were expected (especially single mothers) to fulfill multiple roles as economic providers, caregivers, child bearers and child rearers. At the expense of the women's overall health, these conditions were overlooked because not only did excessive profits accrue to both local and external capitalist forces, but these people also held race and gender biases.

The Moyne Report, by making special note of the work and employment conditions of shop assistants, domestic servants, factory and manual workers, identified the important role performed by women in the agricultural and non-agricultural sectors.[35] However, in general, reports documenting the Caribbean during this time period only give a passing reference to the impact of unemployment and underemployment on the well being of women and the effect their conditions had on their lives and the lives of their children. Williams, in highlighting the plight of children, mentioned that [w]ith the mothers debilitated by hookworm, half-starved and vulnerable to waterborne diseases, the infant mortality rate was staggering.[36]

Construction of health facilities during the pre-independent colonial era was slow and the services remained confined to the welfare of mothers and children and to some public health education measures. In several of the islands, voluntary associations such as child welfare leagues, child welfare associations and maternity leagues were established, mainly by the church; and these generally reflected the extent of the services offered.

The health care sector was not the only one lacking; the provisions made by schools were inadequate and "the education provided was woefully deficient in quality" resulting in extremely high illiteracy rates. The economic situation also continued to deteriorate and the population, to a great extent, survived on the remittances sent home by relatives who had emigrated. However, the channels for emigration for Black Caribbean people to the USA, Panama and Britain became less accessible, and as they did so the protests grew. In 1935, sugar workers in St. Kitts and British Guiana (renamed Guyana after Independence in 1966) went on strike and this was followed by a coal strike against increased custom duties in St. Vincent. In 1937, the oil field workers in Trinidad went on a strike that eventually evolved into a general island-wide strike and, later, its effect was even more widespread causing labour unrest in Barbados, St. Lucia, British Guiana, and Jamaica. The British government reacted by sending military troops into Guyana to support the local police and soldiers; a total of 115 people were wounded in the process, 29 people were killed and considerable damage was done to property.[37] The heightened consciousness of the working-class was also demonstrated by the formation of labour unions throughout the region and the simultaneous emergence of political parties.[38]

To deal with these new developments, the British government sent another commission to the Caribbean. A West Indian Conference was organized to consider the issue of federation and full elective control of the legislative assemblies. The commission was opposed to "the grant of universal adult suffrage until the present standard of education in the islands had greatly advanced,"[39] and the British government was opposed to a federation which would lead to self-government, but saw it as a mechanism which would bring economic benefits and improve administrative efficiency.[40] As a result, "no solution was reached on the question of adult suffrage and each colony was left to work out independent franchise qualifications."[41] It was the general feeling among Caribbean leaders that the British were anxious to make the federation work so that its obligation to the region would be minimized.

The need for a unified Caribbean union went beyond the politicians. Several professional regional associations worked towards having uniformity in education, law and health systems and fighting against racial discrimination in the colonial civil service. When the West Indies Labour Congress met in 1938 in British Guiana, some of the regional demands made to the colonial governments were for federation, a legislature elected through adult suffrage and social legislation such as old age pension, national health insurance, unemployment insurance, minimum wage, 44-hour week, workmen's compensation, trade union immunities, and free, compulsory elementary education.

1940 to 1960

The first Colonial Development and Welfare Act (a consequence of the Moyne Commission), which was passed in 1940, set in place the first organized state health system in the English-speaking Caribbean, committing £500,000 a year from 1940 to 1950 "for social and economic development in the colonies" and a lump sum of £500,000, specifically for research.[42] Sir Frank Stockdale, the first Comptroller for Development and Welfare in the Caribbean, in his 1940-42 report, expressed concern about organizing services that "would promote the health of the whole population" rather than just provide "relief to the poor." Stockdale's proposal visualized the establishment of a "health unit system" in rural areas which would offer small communities similar health services to those provided by larger, more developed urban health centres, but on a much simpler and less costly scale.[43] These health units marked the beginning of a new model of health care within the region; unfortunately, a number of factors retarded their development. These included the lack of experience in the implementation of the "health unit" concept, lack of resources and the time taken in arousing public consciousness in health matters.[44]

However, these systems in modified forms are still in place today and are almost identical in their concept of Primary Health Care systems and centers.

[The] "health unit" system formed the basis for the

extensive network of health services in the Caribbean today and can be called responsible, to a great extent, for the impressive reduction in infant and child mortalities in the Caribbean.[45]

During the 1950s, considerable effort went into controlling endemic diseases such as malaria, hookworm, tuberculosis, small-pox and yaws. Through a combined strategy, which involved the Colonial Development and Welfare Funds, PAHO/WHO, UNICEF and the Rockefeller Foundation, most of the communicable diseases were brought under control.[46] Although very few additional health centres and hospitals were built, efforts were made to improve the quantity and quality of services and to enhance utilization. Greater emphasis was placed on the development of safe water supplies, improved sanitation, slum clearance and enhanced housing.[47] Many of the social and economic issues facing the Caribbean masses were carried over to the independence period.

The abolition of colonialism was the main concern of colonial nationalist movements which were formed around 1942. Nationalism and class consciousness, which took different forms depending on the metropolitan country with which the colonial state was involved,[48] had increased during the period of World War I. Several Caribbean nationals had returned home after military service, and incensed by the racism at home, joined in the fight for change.[49] The local struggle gained confidence from similar protests which were taking place at that same time in the USA (the Civil Rights Movement) and gave the Caribbean middle class an opportunity to make a number of demands. These included: racial equality in the civil service and democratic institutions, widening the franchise, reforming the constitution and seeking federation of the islands.

A series of developments occurred in several of the larger islands. Jamaica achieved adult suffrage in 1944, followed by Trinidad two years later. A ministerial system of government was introduced and the discussions for the proposed regional federation commenced. While these talks were in process, the Constitution of the Guyana Government was suspended in 1953 by the British Government on the alleged grounds that the People's Progressive Party (PPP) was planning to introduce a communist state; and in neighbouring Trinidad a new "democratic" political party (the People's National Movement (PNM)) emerged. The Federation established in 1958 collapsed in 1962, a break-up attributed to a number of factors including lack of involvement of working class people in the process and dependency of Caribbean politicians on the colonial government for guidance and decision making.

POST-COLONIALISM/INDEPENDENCE (1960 to 1980)

By the 1960s, some of the larger Caribbean countries had gained political independence: Jamaica and Trinidad and Tobago in 1962, Guyana and Barbados in 1966. The smaller countries like Grenada had graduated to an internal self-government but had to wait until the 1970s to become independent states. Within the region, the US replaced Britain as the major outside influence and economic financier. Lewis noted that Jamaica, Trinidad and Tobago and Barbados, "although they remained members of the British Commonwealth.... became increasingly dependent upon the US for trade and financial aid."[50]

Independence saw the rapid growth of state ownership and increased control in areas such as the social sector where there were provisions of new and improved welfare services including health, education, community development, old age pension and national insurance. The policies developed by government did not change the social structure of the society but adapted colonial models to fit into the existing new politically independent nations. Thomas argued that the social services introduced were minimal in range and, in fact, no policies were advocated which tackled poverty as a social problem. He stated that implicit in this approach was the assumption that the benefits of economic growth would eventually trickle down to the poor and so ensure the development of the whole society.[51]

However, unemployment problems in the 1960s remained acute, reaching 20 per cent in Jamaica and 15 per cent in Trinidad and Tobago. The rate was particularly high among the 15-25 age group and was higher among women than men.[52] Emigration became the main outlet for economic survival[53], especially for young (20-34 years old) skilled and semi-skilled men although a large number of unskilled labourers also migrated. This created a gender imbalance in the population that is still reflected in the present unequal female/male ratios that exist in most Caribbean countries and accounts for the large "female-headed" household phenomena within the Caribbean (about 70% of all births occur to unmarried women and approximately 33% of households, on average, are headed by women[54]). For women, this meant that they continued to form the bulk of the labour force, working in large numbers in low paying jobs as agriculture labourers, street vendors, and as domestics in households. They also formed the backbone of the education and health sector, employed as teachers and nurses. Generally, more women in the society became solely responsible for the economic as well as emotional well-being of their families.

The political, social and economic progress made in the post-colonial period contributed towards the improvements of the health and living standards of the region's population. The first Five Year Development Plan from an independent Caribbean country came out of Jamaica in 1962. The Plan placed great emphasis on providing clean water supplies, and immunization programs; facilitating the modernization of hospital facilities and the decentralization of the management of hospitals, health centres and dispensaries; and ensuring the proper financial administration at the central level of the Ministry of Health. Similar developments also took place in other larger independent countries, but were much slower in the smaller territories. The implementation of these public health measures generally increased the health of the population at large, as is reflected in the increase in life expectancy throughout the region. (See Table 5.1)

During the late 1960s and the 1970s, most governments spent significant portions of their revenue on education, health and other social services. For example, Trinidad and Tobago's 15 Year Development Plan 1968 to 1983 was targeted to spend on education $171 million dollars (TNT) in capital expenditure ($1,144 million dollars (TNT) in recurrent expenditure).[55] The government also proposed to increase free secondary education (started in 1960) in order to cover 91 percent of the twelve to fourteen (12-14) year age group.[56] With the establishment of state health policies within the region, priority was placed on the training and re-training of health personnel. The University of the

West Indies, School of Public Health, PAHO/WHO and several other national and international organizations contributed to the training of a large number of doctors, nurses, midwives, auxiliary nurses, public health nurses, public health inspectors, nutritionists, health educators and laboratory technicians. Services were primarily focused on mothers and children, and concentrated on birth and early childhood. Ante-natal care was started very early in the pregnancy and care continued after birth. Traditional midwives were replaced by hospital-trained and based midwives who were responsible for delivering over 90 percent of all babies born in 1980.[57] However, all this was done within the existing context of a responsive medical model of care without equal expansion and promotion of a preventative model.

Table 5.1
Life Expectancy at Birth (years) by Country, Region and Sex 1965-1975 and 1975-1980

Country	1965-1975		1975-1980	
	Men	**Women**	**Men**	**Women**
Barbados	65.1	70.8	67.6	72.5
Guyana	65.2	67.5	66.5	71.7
Jamaica	65.9	69.7	67.8	72.5
Trinidad & Tobago	65.9	69.7	65.2	72.0
The Caribbean	58.8	62.4	60.2	64.8

Source: Beckles, Gloria, "The Health of Women in the English-speaking Caribbean: Mortality Rates, Cardiovascular Diseases and Cancers," 1992, p.15.

This chapter outlined the circumstances under which Caribbean women lived and the consequences of those conditions on their health. The following chapters on Barbados and Grenada will examine in detail several aspects of women's political and socio-economic development as a way of understanding the policy decisions made in relationship to the development of health services received by women.

Most countries in the region, including Barbados and Grenada (prior to 1979) had health care systems that were based on the British model and represented three different levels of care: Primary (basic services, health education, preventative care), Secondary (acute care) and Tertiary care (chronic/long term). Whether the models adopted by Barbados and Grenada were appropriate, or were appropriately adapted, for the delivery of Primary Health Care in these countries and whether they were implemented to the benefit of women, particularly working class women, will be reviewed. The reviews are done through the detailed examination of two Caribbean countries, Barbados and Grenada both of which implemented PHC models using different strategies with resulting different outcomes. Barbados used the British National Health System Model and Grenada, the Alma Ata Primary Health Care model with socialist influences.

Notes

1. Lewis, Gordon, K. *Main Currents in Caribbean Thought: The Historical Evolution of Caribbean in its Ideological Aspects, 1492-1900*: 1983: p. 5. See also Williams (1970), Beckles (1990), Parry and Sherlock (1956).
2. Issac Dookhan. *A Pre-Emancipation History of the West Indies*: Longman Caribbean, 1971:14.
3. Ibid see also Knight (1978); Williams (1970).
4. Olive Senior *Working Miracles: Women's Lives in the English-Speaking Caribbean*. Cave Hill, Barbados: ISER, University of the West Indies, 1991:106.
5. RS. Sheridan. *Sugar and Slavery: An Economic History of the British West Indies*: Caribbean University Press, 1985:341.
6. Shaheen Ali "Making the Shift from Multicultural Health to Anti-Racist Health" *Healthbeat,* 12:3: Ontario Public Health Association, Summer 1993 :6.
7. Ibid.
8. Ibid.
9. Cecilia Green (1992): 36.
10. Shaeen Ali (1993).
11. See Gordon K Lewis. *Main Currents in Caribbean Thought*: the Historical Evolution of Caribbean Society in its Ideological Aspects 1492-1900:John Hopkins University Press, 1983.
12. See RS. Sheridan (1985).
13. Hilary Beckles (1990).
14. Free Blacks were former slaves who achieved their freedom either, at the discretion of their masters, after either serving more than twenty years (those referred to in the text probably attained their

freedom this way), or by escaping and retreating to the mountains (as did the Maroons in Jamaica, 1734, and the Bush Negroes in Surinam, 1728) See Eric Williams (1970).

15. R S. Sheridan (1985).
16. Lucille Mathurin "The Rebel Woman in the British West Indies During Slavery." Jamaica: The African Caribbean Institute, 1975.
17. See R.S. Sheridan (1985).
18. JH. Parry and P.M.Sherlock. *A Short History of the West Indies*. London: Macmillian & Co Ltd, 1970:183.
19. JH. Parry and P.M. Sherlock (1970).
20. See Hilary Beckles (1990).
21. Eric Williams *From Columbus to Castro: The History of the Caribbean 1492-1969* London: Andre Deutsch Ltd, 1970:328
22. Ibid.:329.
23. See JH. Parry and P.M. Sherlock, 1970.
24. Lord Stanley, the sponsor of the Emancipation Act admitted in 1848 that the apprenticeship period was in effect "modified slavery" (quoted by Williams Eric, 1970):331-328.
25. See Eric Williams (1970).
26. The illegitimate off-spring of plantation owners and Black ex/slaves were referred to as "Coloureds."
27. See RS. Sheridan (1985).
28. JH. Parry and P.M. Sherlock (1970).
29. See Clive Y Thomas. *The Poor and the Powerless: Economic Policy and Change in the Caribbean*: Latin American Bureau, 1988.
30. See Olive Senior (1991).
31. See Jocelyn Massiah (1986), also see Hilary Beckles (1990)
32. Eric Williams (1970):331.
33. The Moyne Report which documented the underlying socio-economic causes of the uprisings, was released in 1948 see Eric Williams (1970).
34. Clive Y Thomas. *The Poor and the Powerless: Economic Policy and Change in the Caribbean*: Latin American Bureau, 1988:50 see also Ferguson (1990); Williams (1970); Knight (1978) and Lewis (1968).
35. See Eric Williams (1970):444.
36. Ibid.:449.
37. See Olive Senhor (1991):109.
38. Eric Williams (1970):454.
39. See Franklin W Knight (1978).
40. Several political parties were formed in the late 30s and early 40s, including: the Oilfield Workers Union in Trinidad (1937), the British Guiana Labour Union (1937), the Bustamante Industrial Trade Union in Jamaica (1938), and the Barbados Workers Union

(1941). The Windward Islands were late in starting trade unions (only St. Vincent had a union formed before 1945) and it was not until 1950 that the Grenada Manual and Mental Workers Union was formed. See Franklin W. Knight (1987):119. See also Issac Dookan (1975): 93-97.

41. Eric Williams (1970):474.
42. See Gordon K Lewis (1968):345.
43. Eric Williams (1970): 474; See also Gordon Lewis (1968)
44. Dinesh Sinha (1988):125.
45. See Dinesh Sinha (1988).
46. Ibid.:224.
47. Ibid.:126.
48. Ibid.
49. Ibid.:128.
50. See Eric Williams (1970).
51. Clive Thomas (1988), Franklin W Knight (1978).
52. James Ferguson (1990):20.
53. Clive Y Thomas (1988):196.
54. Eric Williams (1990).
55. Nearly 15 million West Indians left for greener pastures between 1950 and 1980. Some 725,000 people emigrated from Jamaica, 204,000 from Trinidad & Tobago, 187,000 from Guyana, 73,000 from Barbados and 52,000 from Grenada. See Dinesh Sinha (1988), see also Eric Williams (1970) and Jack Harewood (1984).
56. See Dorian Powell (1986), see also Dinesh Sinha (1988) and Jocelyn Massiah (1982).
57. See Williams (1970):476.
58. Ibid.
59. See Jeanette Bell (1992).

CHAPTER 6

BARBADOS

THE POLITICAL SITUATION

Prior to 1979

Established in 1938 in response to the 1937 workers' rebellion, the Barbados Labour Party (BLP) was the first political party to be formed in post colonial Barbados. The Party was described by Beckles as "a political organization designed to provide political expression for the island's law abiding inhabitants."[1] This distinction was made in order to dissociate the Party's image from the radical politics of Clement Payne, a leader in the 1937 workers' rebellion whose followers and supporters were described by the State as the "lawless" poor. The BLP, which subsequently changed its name to the Barbados Progressive League (BPL), was "essentially a middle-class led organization vying for a mass base in order to confront and eventually reduce the oligarchic political power of the consolidated merchant-planter elite."[2]

Sir Grantley Adams, a so called "gradualist reformer, the colonial moderate," became leader of the BPL by using a combination of strategies. Internally he got the support of the local plantocracy by convincing them that "legislative concessions to the working masses was in their long-term interests"[3] and got rid of Party members who opposed him. Externally he received the support of the colonial office by successfully assuring the Moyne Commission in 1939 "that neither he nor his colleagues were communists or supporters of such organizations, but socialists committed to an equitable distribution of economic resources and the liberation of social institutions...."[4] Sir Grantley Adams also became President of The Barbados Workers Union (BWU) which developed out of BPL committees and was appointed by the union to address the issue "of workers compensation and the process of legalising wage agreements."[5]

In 1946 the League resorted to its original name, the Barbados Labour Party, and by 1951 had succeeded in winning the elections (by a small majority) and becoming the ruling government. The victory gave Sir Grantley Adams, who remained "conservative and pro-British," the power to purge the BLP and the BWU of "radical elements."[6] Errol Barrow (then a BLP member) resigned before Adams could ask him to leave and in 1955 formed the Democratic Labour Party (DLP) which consisted of several progressive former members of the BLP and BWU.

The BLP leadership was considered "the vehicle of colonial socialism" not only on the domestic scene but also at the regional level. Adams and his administration cut links with the Caribbean Labour Council (CLC), "the chief instrument of the communist front-organization in the area,"[7] and in particular with two of the known Marxist members, Dr. Cheddie Jagan of Guyana (presently President of Guyana) and Richard Hart of Jamaica.

From 1954 to 1961 the Barbados Labour Party, with the assistance of Barbados Workers Union (BWU), developed what was described as "the rudimentary welfare state of contemporary Barbados."[8] Several pieces of legislation and social reforms were put into place; these included a guaranteed daily wage for sugar workers, the Labour Welfare Fund, a workman's compensation scheme, holiday with pay, and the 44-hour work week.[9] The BWU was especially instrumental in championing the cause of the working class and in particular "helped give a new status to the working class woman" in the fight for better wages for shop assistants. However there was a feeling that, although both the Union and Party had made changes which improved the lives of workers, these changes were merely "ameliorative" and "no fundamental reshaping of the structure of society"[10].The Democratic Labour Party defeated the BLP at the 1961 parliamentary elections and Errol Barrow went on to become the longest ruling Barbadian Prime Minister (1961 to 1976), leading his nation into independence in 1966. Barrow's views were remarkably different from Adam's as he

> opposed the invasion of a single piece of English-speaking society by forces of the United States. Of equal logic and force was his unrelenting insistence that the Caribbean should be a zone of peace and not an area for ever-increasing penetration by foreign forces, from whatever source and however cunningly disguised.[11]

One of Barrow's first major national achievements was the introduction of free secondary education in the public school system. In January, 1962; and later, in 1963, the DLP administration was also instrumental in the local establishment of the Cave Hill Campus of the University of the West Indies which included the regional Faculty of Law. These openings in the educational system gave children of working class parentage an opportunity to receive higher education, to excel and eventually to hold senior positions within the society.

Barrow was not only a strong proponent of national development, but also of regional unity and integration and saw "economic integration as the only viable framework within which economic development could be pursued."[12] He was instrumental in the formation of several regional agencies such as the establishment of the Caribbean Free Trade Association (CARIFTA,1968; now the Caribbean Common Market or CARICOM), the Caribbean Development Bank (1970) and the Caribbean Community (1970).

Ideologically, the BLP and the DLP are very similar, a feature that has contributed to the high level of post-independence political stability on Barbados, and has been attributed to:

> the broad consensus between the two major parties on economic and national policies and the accommodation between the black middle class, who control party

politics, and the rich whites, who own the wealth of the country and represent an exclusive, racially separatist economic elite. A division of labour has evolved in which the white minority dominates the ownership of capital while the black middle class moves in the centres of elite power by way of professions. Both groups cohere in political coalitions and share power over decision-making but remain apart on the social level. This balance of forces could easily be overturned if the blacks began to demand more control over the economy and less racial and social exclusivity within the elite, but the ideological trends in Barbados politics are not yet moving in that direction.[13]

Thus, despite its newly acquired sovereignty, Barbados continued to be ruled by an entrenched Westminster-style government which, as Beckles argued:

was perhaps inevitable given the absence of political activity within the ruling Democratic Labour Party, or the opposition Barbados Labour Party, which sought to distance the island from the institutional and constitutional structures inherited during the colonial era....Independence within the confines of the imperial Commonwealth system was what the Democratic Labour Party government had proposed and attained in 1966, and the rejection of republicanism, in itself a popular measure, was perhaps the most obvious indicator of the limits which would be placed upon nationalism thereafter. The appointment of the last imperial Governor as the first Governor-General of the free state was also symbolic of the gradualist and moderate nature of the transition implied by constitutional independence.[14]

The island still maintains a two-party political culture in which the BLP and DLP, collectively, have a hegemonic claim over the electorate.

The 1979 to 1983 Period

Tom Adams (Sir Grantley Adam's son), now leader of the Barbados Labour Party, won the 1976 parliamentary election. The victory was attributed to a shift in priorities from the social problems facing their countries to the external economic pressures it was experiencing. The mid-1970s economic crisis which increased the international price of oil,

> resulted in a premium being placed upon financial and managerial acumen within regional politics, rather than radical socio-cultural dynamism; this context was effectively exploited by the Barbados Labour Party in the 1976 elections.. with an undoubtedly private-sector image was able to defeat the Democratic Labour Party and restore the sagging confidences of the corporate elite within the country's polity.[15]

Tom Adams' political views (like his father's) were highly conservative, both at home and regionally. His involvement in various activities "reconfirmed the party's image as opposed to socialist decolonisation."[16] In December 1979, the BLP administration assisted the government of St. Vincent by sending in armed forces to recapture Union Island (a dependency of St. Vincent) from "Rastafarian elements." In the same year, James Callaghan, the British government's labour leader, (after attending the summit meeting of the western leaders in the French Caribbean island of Guadeloupe) made a surprise two day visit to Barbados for talks with Prime Minister Tom Adams. The meeting, which was convened with the knowledge of the American government, was organized to persuade other Caribbean governments to develop a mobile regional defence force capable of intervening in any of the Caribbean Contingency Joint Task Force member islands.[17] According to Ambursley & Dunkerley,

> the main target was the government of Barbados, richest of the small islands and the proposed headquarters for the force....Tom Adams had already discussed the idea of the regional force with the St. Lucia leader, John Compton and Callaghan found a receptive audience for his proposal.[18]

Tom Adams and the BLP administration also took a leading "role in gaining the regional isolation of Grenada's socialist revolution in 1979"[19] and worked diligently with other like-minded political leaders in supporting and assisting the U.S. government's invasion of Grenada in 1983. Although Barbados, and most of the other larger More Developed Countries (MDCs)[20] formally recognized the PRG, the smaller Lesser Developed Countries (LDCs) collectively made a decision against formal recognition "fearing that the kind of example of the Bishop model could give rise to "revolutionary elements" in their own states."[21] Adams' ideological position was, however, more in keeping with the sentiments of the smaller states and he became "a leading critic of Marxist and radical political formations in the region."[22] His pro-capitalist stance also greatly influenced the way economic decisions were made by the BLP administration and drove the socio-economic and political relationships with others in and outside of the region.

THE ECONOMIC SITUATION
Prior to 1979

The Barbados economy, an open economy since independence, has diversified away from its traditional sugar base and is now heavily dependent on tourism and, to a lesser extent, manufacturing. During the 1960s and early 1970s, the economy enjoyed significance growth:

> between 1964 and 1971 the annual growth was 11.5 per cent and from 1956 until 1976 the estimated annual growth was as high as 9.5 per cent. In 1964 the per capita national income was about 60 per cent higher than it was in 1956; and between 1953 and 1971 Barbados had the highest per capita national income growth in the West Indies. By 1971 Barbados was second to Trinidad & Tobago (an oil-based economy) who recorded a higher per capita income but it was less than 10 per cent higher.[23]

Although growth took place in the economic sectors of tourism, sugar and manufacturing, high unemployment figures indicated that "rapid growth had failed to deliver the all-round development the authorities had anticipated. The percentage of the labour force unemployed in 1960 and 1965 was just over 12 and 15 per cent respectively. In 1970, the figure was somewhat reduced, but was still quite high at 9 per cent."[24] The lack of any significant decline in the unemployment rate was due in part to the seasonal nature of the dominant economic sectors and other environmental factors, but also to the laissez-faire attitude of Caribbean governments that "allowed employment/unemployment to take care of itself, to remain a by-product of the growth in incomes and output. No systematic attack on unemployment as a high priority has been ever mounted."[25]

From 1973 onward, the economy began to be troubled by inflation, unemployment and the balance of payments.

> During 1974 to 1978 current price of the Gross Domestic Product (GDP) at factor cost exhibited fairly strong growth of 10% per annum on average, rising from $640.4m. in 1974 to $937.3m. in 1978. However, in real terms the average growth rates were very modest at just over 2% per annum, with 1974 and 1975 registering negative real economic growth. Subsequently, there was some measure of recovery with real growth rates of 4.3%, 2.6% and 3.0% in 1976, 1977 and 1978 respectively.[26]

The slight increase in growth rates from 1976 to 1978 were however relatively insignificant and the unemployment rate continued to be quite high. In order to deal with the economic situation in 1978, the BLP put forward a short term economic strategy that included monetary and credit policy, fiscal restraint, selective import control, and incomes and prices policy as measures to cope with four economic problems:[27] (1) the deficit on current account, which they claimed could not be "eliminated immediately merely by increasing the levels of taxation, but only after fundamental structural changes relating to government expenditure patterns, as well as to the tax base"; (2) the balance of payment deficit, which they feared, "based on the 1976/1977 experience....may deplete the country's foreign reserves, with attendant disruptive effects"; (3) the high unemployment rate; and (4) the high inflation.

McLean praised the 1978 budget speech as the "most analytical and clearly articulated Budget Speech ever made in the Barbadian Parliament by a Minister of Finance"; but was nevertheless critical of the BLP's understanding of the main economic problems, claiming that:

> [t]he problem of low wages among a substantial portion of the labour force was not given explicit recognition....There was overemphasis on the prospect of locally generated inflation, and a failure to appreciate the fact that a small open economy must accommodate itself to, rather than resist import-propelled inflation....The imminence of a balance of payments deficit depleting foreign reserves had been exaggerated.... These perceptional deficiencies are also reflected in misplaced emphasis on an Incomes and Prices Policy as a central plank of Government's short-term economic policy. The emphasis on an Incomes and Prices Policy results partly from a failure to accord priority to bringing about a redistribution of income away from profits to wages, as well as a misunderstanding of the actual and potential causes of balance of payments deficit in the Barbadian economy.[28]

1979 to 1983

However, in spite of rising prices of fuel and other imported goods and the increasing economic difficulties of its main trading partners, in the late 1970s Barbados experienced some relief. The Barbados Development Bank's Annual Report 1979 to 1980 claimed that the country had recorded its fourth successive year of real increase in Gross Domestic Produce (GDP). In 1979 the GDP increased by 6.9 percent over the 1978 figure, compared with an average of about 4 percent for the period 1976 to 1978. Real wages increased in almost all sectors of the economy from 1976 to 1980 and unemployment decreased from 15.5 percent in 1976 to 12.6 percent in 1980[29] (this was still above the rate recorded for 1970). Fields argues that the increase in real wages and accompanied decrease in employment were indicators, albeit indirect evidence,[30] that economic growth did help the Barbados labour force.

The growth spurt was, however, short lived and, during 1981, the real GDP declined from BDS $804 million in 1980 to $783 million (a 2.6 percent drop). "It was the first time in six years that negative growth was experienced in the domestic economy, which was severely affected by the recession in the economies of major trading partners."[31] The BLP reported that unemployment by mid 1982 had reached 15 percent, in contrast to the 11 percent level reported for the first half of 1981.[32] High unemployment rates were not limited to Barbados but were experienced throughout the region; in fact the rate was lower in Barbados than in most of the other countries. (See Table 6.1)

Table 6.1
Rate of Unemployment, 1982
(Selected Caribbean Countries)

Country	Rate of Unemployment
Antigua Barbuda	20.0
Barbados	13.6
Belize	14.3*
Dominica	15.0
Grenada	14.2
Jamaica	27.4
Montserrat	5.6
St. Christopher-Nevis	26.0*
St. Lucia	27.0
St. Vincent & the Grenadines	20.0
Trinidad & Tobago	10.4

* 1980 Figures,
Source: Sinha, Dinesh, P., *Children of the Caribbean 1945 to 1984: Progress in Child Survival, its Determinants and Implications,* 1988, p. 54.

With these low employment levels and the export constraints being experienced, productivity in Barbados suffered. In 1982, Barbados saw its sugar output fall below 90,000 tonnes (the worst since 1948); the tourism sector showed little signs of recovery; the manufacturing sector was still plagued by factory closures and staff retrenchments; and the government continued to restrict various credits, virtually freezing loans for such items as cars and mortgages.

Haniff noted that "an important element in the government strategy for recovery of the economy appeared to be restraint on wages, an element which put it in confrontation with the traditionally staid trade unions of Barbados."[33] With the high unemployment levels and signs of labour unrest, the government in 1982 introduced the Unemployment Benefit Scheme and the Emergency Powers Bill.[34] The Unemployment Benefit Scheme helped to cushion the shock by providing assistance to a number of workers, mainly older persons who lost their jobs. The Emergency Bill, which gave government the power to prevent strikes, was not popular and received objections from opposition members and trade unions on the grounds that it gave excessive and wide powers to the minister. Since the government gave no reasons for the introduction of the Bill, civil servants who were demanding higher wages, assumed that the Bill was directed to them and tensions between the union and the BLP continued to grow.

In defence of the poorly performing economy (the decline of output and income and the increase in unemployment), Tom Adams pointed to the recession and the restrictions major trading partners placed on their import levels. "The result was that the export-oriented sectors were considerably weakened."[35] During 1983, unemployment figures increased (by 2,300 persons from the 1981 figure) to 14,900 persons; 6,400 (43%) of which were males and 8,500 (or 57%) were females; and 8,000 (more than 50%) were under the age of 25 (only 1,600 were over 40 years old). "This clearly indicates that the thrust of the government's effort to generate employment must continue to be geared towards matching a supply of jobs with the needs of the young and relatively unskilled, especially female, segment of the labour force."[36]

The government did, however, make a few concessions over the 1979 to 1983 period in order to alleviate the financial burden people were facing. These included the abolition of charges for school meals (1979); increases in the non-contributory Old Age Pension Plan for persons 65 and over (1979); payments of additional money and free public transportation between scheduled hours were made available to pensioners; and the Unemployment Benefit Scheme (1982) which provided assistance to a number of persons who lost their jobs, "mainly older workers who could more easily qualify under the present stringent conditions."[37]

Tom Adam's regime managed to stay in power from 1976 to 1985 despite the serious economic and social problems that confronted them, and in spite of popular criticism that the government was principally concerned with "white elite interests and the defence of American imperialist strategies within the region"[38] and not with the issues facing working class peoples, including those specifically facing working class women.

THE STATE AND WOMEN
Prior to 1979

[A]lthough the status of women has been elevated in the twentieth century and particularly in the last thirty years, the attitudes of a male dominated society are still affected by the past; the law of the eighteenth century has been radically altered but the customs and attitudes of that age have died harder and in some cases not at all.[39]

Despite the fact that Barbadian women received the vote in 1943, few women were elevated to positions of political power. For example, even though the 1960s saw more women as senators, the proportion of female to male senators remained very small. Of the twelve government senators, only one was a woman; and of the seven independent senators, two were women. Only one woman was elected to the House of Assembly (in 1976) and only two women were appointed to the Legislative Assembly (now Senate), a BLP candidate from 1951 to 1961, and a DLP candidate and Parliamentary Secretary from 1971 to 1976. Only one woman has ever held a ministerial position (1976 to 1985) during the BLP administration. (The DLP as of 1992 still had not appointed any women to ministerial rank.) The advances women made in politics and also in business were small when compared to those advances made in education although in reality only a small proportion of Barbadian women benefited from the educational opportunities.

One of the major accomplishments of the Tom Adams' administration was no doubt the establishment of a National Commission on the Status of Women (NCSW) in November 1976. This originated out of an appeal made by "Women in Action", a NGO coalition, for government to establish a department or bureau that would be headed by a woman and adequately staffed to deal specifically with women's affairs, including research into women's legal status and the position of women in important sectors, vis-à-vis men. This recommendation was reviewed and, in March 1976, the House of Assembly passed a resolution to establish a Commission mandated to inquire into the status of women. The Commission then proposed the establishment of a Women's Bureau that would initially act as its Secretariat; both units were established simultaneously and located within the parent Ministry, Legal Affairs.[40]

The Commission collected data previously unavailable on the status of women in Barbados and, in May 1978, presented a two volume report to Henry Forde, the Minister responsible for Women's Affairs (and then Attorney General). The Report stated that since the formation of the Barbados Labour Party (BLP) in 1938, a record of 110 women had served on the National Executive Council up to the year 1978; a number of women also served on the National Executive Council of the Democratic Labour Party (DLP) which was founded in 1955, but no exact figures were available. Only one woman had attained ambassadorial rank and held the post from 1975 to 1976. The appointments to Statutory Boards and the Board of Management of Codrington College revealed the same inequities: three woman were appointed Chairs of Boards and three Deputy Chairs; on the 57 Boards, there were 327 men and 67 women, a ratio of almost 5 to 1. It was noted that the Child Care Board, which at the time was comprised of 7 women (the Deputy Chair being a woman) and 3 men, was the only one on which a large number of women were represented. The Film Censorship Board also had a larger representation of women; there were 6 women and 4 men. Thus, Norma Forde noted that "... Barbadian women are not usually appointed to head those bodies which relate to business corporations and financial institutions."[41]

In presenting the Report, which contained 212 recommendations and covered six areas (law, employment, education, health, family and miscellaneous) to Parliament in September 1987, Minister Henry Forde expressed the hope that "in the pursuit of the policy of true equality of the sexes and in seeking to give women in Barbados a new deal, the government would take all necessary steps to implement at the earliest opportunity, the Commission's recommendations."[42]

1979 to 1983

In 1979 Norma Forde, then Chair of the Commission, carried out an assessment of the progress made in the implementation of the Commission recommendations and reported that some of the recommendations had received attention. For example, sixteen of the forty-six recommendations in relation to the law had been effected by legislation making provision for the proposed changes. The laws which were given parliamentary approval included: the Marriage Act; the Domicile Reform Act; the Status of Children Reform Act; the Property Act; and separate income tax assessment for husbands and wives. Much discussion, with promises of relevant statutory changes, had also taken place on improvement of community services, problems associated with employment and unemployment, and the kind of expansion needed to create new jobs. Concern for mental and physical health was also evident in the proposed National Health Legislation and its services.

However, despite these noted improvements in the status of women, Norma Forde argued that:

> [i]mportant areas have been left untouched. The law relating to rape needs reorganizing; maintenance of women both in and out of wedlock is still rigidly prescribed, procedurally protracted and in some cases legally non-existent. Judicial separation and divorce proceedings are subjected to unwarranted delays resulting in hardships often to both parties but chiefly to women. A proposal for an Indecency with Children Act remains a proposal. The legal aid scheme is still being discussed. Altogether there is a general lack of

urgency to this kind of social law reform ... A recommendation was made for constituting a Status of Women Council as an independent body with the authority to initiate and monitor programs relating to women. There is no evidence that this recommendation has been effected. The Report includes useful information which could have been disseminated by all sections of the media. Regrettably this has not been done.[43]

Gillings also observed that, although Barbadian women had benefited from bold and imaginative family law reforms and appeared to be enjoying improved socio-economic status (compared with other Caribbean women), there were still many contradictions:

While there are many legal reforms, many women are unaware of their legal rights; despite high educational levels they are still experiencing high unemployment; they continue to participate unequally with men in the areas of vocational skill training, concentrating in a narrow range of skills and occupational areas; they are still physically abused; they do not participate equally in the boardrooms; despite the fact that over 50% of voters are women, they are lowly represented in the decision-making levels in politics with a similar situation in the public service.[44]

The Bureau which had began functioning on its own (without NCSW) in 1978, was transferred to the Ministry of Labour and Community Services and remained there from May 1979 to 81. Another move, to Transport, Works and Community Service, occurred during 1981 to 1982 and yet another during 1982 to 1985, this time to Information and Culture. During the period 1979 to 1983, the Bureau had not only changed ministers three times but also ministries; these moves, which must have interrupted the growth and development of the Bureau, reflected the lack of importance given to women's affairs by government. (Note during the period after the study time frame and up to the time of this research, the Bureau had moved twice more. From 1985 to 1991, the Bureau was located in Employment, Labour Relations and Community Development, and from November 1992 to present, in the Ministry of Housing, Land, Community and Culture.) It was therefore not surprising to find that since 1976, three different women occupied the post of acting director and that the position was only filled in 1984.

According to Norma Forde, the Commission had visualized the Division of Women's Affairs as a vibrant, well-organized unit and had recommended that the present Bureau be extended and strengthened; however, she found no available evidence of this reorganization. In a review of the Bureau in 1987, Gillings noted that its objectives also could not be found in the records of Cabinet or civil service establishment. In fact the Bureau was presently functioning on the original mandate adopted by Parliament in 1976 that proposed "the establishment of a Women's Bureau which would serve initially as the Secretariat for the Commission."[45] She claimed that the objectives were however imbedded in various documents and emerged only as the Bureau began to function on its own:[46]

- Monitor generally the situation relating to women;
- Keep track of the recommendations made by the NCSWC and to ensure that these are implemented;
- Make recommendations concerning matters which affect women;
- Undertake consciousness raising activities in the community on the role of women;
- Identify projects;
- Promote research about the problems and needs of women and disseminate the results;
- Create and maintain linkages with Government, regional and international agencies concerned with women's issues.

According to Gillings however, the above objectives represented additional and expanded functions to the Bureau's original mandate and these had not (as of 1987) been formally accepted.[47]

Gillings noted that although the Bureau had carried out a series of public education programmes which received full public participation there was concern "about the limited follow-up; there are hardly any reports of the outcomes or examples of the Bureau being able to identify or promote project ideas and programmes as a result of such efforts."[48] The failure of the Bureau to carry out these activities was blamed on inadequate staff. Gillings further criticized the inadequate monitoring functions undertaken by the Bureau in making sure that the Commission's recommendations were implemented, but noted that this was not unique to Barbados and was also a problem experienced by other national machineries in the region as a result of scarce resources. She was also astute in pointing out that although the Economic Affairs Division of the Ministry of Finance maintained linkages with the current host Ministry on development issues pertaining to certain sectors, there was an absence of dialogue on issues specific to women in development. The Five-Year National Development Plan, coordinated and published by Economic Affairs, does not include issues on women's affairs, and projects' analyses carried out by the Division did not take into consideration gender issues.[34] Gillings was also unable to find any reports of the Bureau being invited to, or ever being a member on boards, committees or task forces of any key sectors such as tourism, industry, information, or training. For example, the Bureau was by-passed when the host ministry appointed a task force to examine measures to generate employment in Barbados and women's interest. Representation on behalf of women was made by the National Organization of Women (NOW). The absence of the Bureau at these decision making and planning levels reveals the lack of commitment the government had in addressing "gender discrimination and inequality" and other women's concerns as an area of priority.

Gillings however failed to examine the advocacy role being played by the Bureau in relation to critical concerns of women. For example the Abortion Law, which decriminalized Abortion in 1978, had liberalized the ancient law relating to abortion which was under the historic Offenses Against the Person Act of 1861. The Act prohibited the administration of drugs or the use of instruments to procure abortion anytime after the conception of the child. It was not until 1983 that the government after much debate passed the controversial Medical Termination Pregnancy Act. This was a welcomed piece of legislation, especially for poor women who generally were the ones exposed to illegal abortions. The Act, however, fell short of giving women control over their own bodies and ended up transferring more power and control to the medical establishment. It stipulated that in order for a woman to receive a legal abortion after 12 weeks, she must make a written declaration that "she reasonably believed that her pregnancy was caused by an act of rape or incest and is sufficient to constitute the element of grave injury to her physical and mental health."[50] Thus, although the Act in itself was a progressive piece of legislation it was nevertheless limited, and as of 1992 the Act had not been reviewed. The Bureau has, therefore, been lax in giving the issue the kind of attention that is needed.

Gillings may also have been unaware that the Director of the Bureau's position is a political appointment and that once the BLP lost power to the DLP in 1986, the incumbent Director of the Bureau was viewed as such by the new administration, and was consequently replaced. The concerns of women were, therefore, made secondary by the ruling elite and to the "masculinist dominance" of the State. [51] The fact that the functioning of the Bureau was reduced to the level of partisan loyalties is grounds for making the case that the concerns of women were placed secondary to the interest of government. Women at all socio-economic levels need to be empowered and given the opportunity/right to make informed decisions about issues affecting their lives. Clearly what is needed in Barbados is a body that would collectively convey and advocate the concerns of women. Norma Forde highlighted this systemic deficiency when she noted that:

> [a] strong Department would need the kind of authority and expertise not presently included. Women are daily confronted by specific, serious problems and there is no agency which combines the necessary impartiality and expertise backed by the authoritative credibility necessary to assist them beneficially. [52]

THE HEALTH CARE SYSTEM
Health Infrastructure

Barbados' health care system at first glance can be described as well organized and managed; however, a closer look reveals it to be fragmented. As with other systems in the region, health care in Barbados is stratified into three levels (Primary Health Care (PHC), Secondary Health Care (SHC), and Tertiary Health Care) (THC); and operates on a 2-tier system, with services being provided by both the public and private sector. Each sector is independently financed and as a result there is heavy competition for control over the provision of services and the consistency in quality is lacking.

The Ministry of Health is the chief provider of public health services and is under the directorship of the Minister who reports directly to and is held accountable to the Cabinet. The government health sector is financed primarily by general revenue and a 2% levy which is divided between employer and employee. In addition, user fees are collected at the hospital, for laboratory, X-ray and drug services. The public sector is also responsible for providing services (X-ray and laboratory) through the government hospital, to the private sector.

(Recently more of these services are being provided by the private sector through privately owned medical facilities).

The private medical sector, which has no statutory responsibility, provides predominantly curative services and some maternal and child health services. Medical care is carried out by general practitioners and specialists providing full-time or part-time "in-office" services on a fee-for-service basis while secondary and tertiary care is provided at two general hospitals: The Queen Elizabeth (Q.E.H) and the St. Joseph's Hospitals (the latter is a privately run institution).[53] Statistics show that Barbadians spend approximately 6% of their personal budgets on health care.[54] This would imply that more use is made of the government services; however, unfortunately, there are no official statistics available on the number of patients seen by these private medical practitioners.[55]

This study focuses mainly on the Primary Health Care (PHC) or the Preventive Services provided by the State during 1979-1983. However, references will also be made, from time to time, to Secondary Health Care (SHC) since the polyclinics also provide this level of care within their local communities. PHC services (including care to the elderly, disadvantaged and those suffering from chronic diseases[56]) were/are delivered through the seven refurbished and upgraded health centres or polyclinics as they are called. (The government at the time had plans to construct a new one in 1987.) SHC and THC were/are provided mainly through the Queen Elizabeth, Psychiatric and Geriatric Hospitals and includes those medical care services which cannot be provided through the polyclinics. Before the advent of the polyclinics, the Queen Elizabeth Hospital, which is the only public acute medical facility, was responsible for much of the primary care services and as such some people still use these services in cases of emergency and when the polyclinics are closed (weekdays after 4pm, weekends and holidays). The map of Barbados shows the location of the polyclinics and other health facilities.

Figure 6.1:
Map of Barbados: Location of Polyclinics and Other Health Facilities

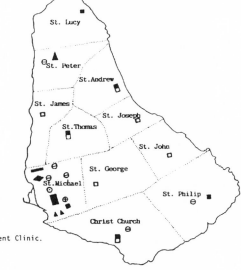

■   Queen Elizabeth Hospital.

■   District Hospital.

◘   District Hospital and Out-patient Clinic.

❑   Out-patient Clinic.

◆   Psychiatric Hospital.

▬   Leprosarium.

▲   St. Joseph's Hospital.

▴   Private Hospital.

⊕   Sir Winston Scott Polyclinic with Laboratory and X-ray Unit.

Θ   Polyclinic: Maurice Byer - St. Peter, Six Roads - St. Philip, Warrens - St. Michael, Black Rock - St. Michael, Edgar Cochrane - St. Michael, Randal Phillips - Christ Church.

Health Care Financing

During 1976 to 1979, the BLP government spent on average 14.1 percent of the combined current and capital account on health care. This figure represented a decrease in expenditure from previous years when government spent an average of 16 percent per year and in 1972 - 73 as much as 17.9 percent [57] This figure was, however, still generally higher than the expenditures of others in the region. For example, Jamaica spent about 12.1 percent of its 1977 to 1978 combined current and capital expenditure on health; health received 10.5 percent of 1978 to 1979 budget.[58]

The level of national expenditure in a particular social service is usually a fair indicator of the importance government attaches to that sector.[59] Using this premise, it may be fair to say that Barbados has placed a high premium on health care. (See Table 6.2 for a breakdown of the Health Budget) However, it is extremely interesting to note that the major portion of the 1983 health budget (and the subsequent estimate for 1983 showed at least 50% of the budget) was allocated to the expansion of the Queen Elizabeth Hospital, a facility which is the main provider of acute medical care. This under-emphasis of PHC is contrary to government's adoption of the Alma Ata Declaration of 1978 and stated commitment "to decentralize medical care as much as possible by the establishment of the PHC through a network of polyclinics which when fully developed should be able to meet more than 80 percent of the demand for health services in the comprehensive health care delivery system."[60] This is not to say that investments were not made in the PHC sector. Actually, in order to build the polyclinics, the government borrowed heavily from international sources, particularly from the Inter-American Development Bank, from whom it received Bds$6.6 million.[61] However, this amount was comparatively smaller than allocations made to THC in general.

Table 6.2:
Breakdown of the Health Budget in Barbados:
1976 to 1983 to the nearest million Barbados dollars.

Financial Period	Total Recurrent Gov.. Exp.	Total Health Budget	% of . Total Exp.	%. Incr. Over Prev. Year	Exp. on Q.E.H.	% Iincr. Over Prev. Year	% Incr. of Total Budget Spent on Q.E.H	% of Total Budget Spent on Psychi- atric Hosp.
1976–1977	255	37.8	16.6	—	16.4	—	43.5	8.3
1977–1978	268	41.2	15.1	9.1	17.8	8.3	43.2	9.2
1978–1979	286	46.9	16.2	13.8	20.0	12.4	42.6	9.1
1979–1980	341	51.1	15.0	8.9	21.2	5.9	41.5	9.2
1980–1981	426	63.1	14.8	23.4	26.6	—	—	5.9
1981–1982	473	98.7	14.7	56.4	29.0	—	—	6.8
1982–1983	528	85.0	14.2*	13.9*	28.6*	—	—	7.1*

* Approved estimates

Sources: (1) 1976 to 1980 data: Dann, Graham, The Quality of Life in Barbados, 1984, p. 149; (2) 1980 to 1983 data: Ministry of Health and National Insurance. Annual Report of the Chief Medical Officer, 1983, p. 56; Ministry of Health; (2) Chief Medical Officer of Health, Annual Report, 1980, p. 138; (3) Chief Medical Officer of Health, Annual Report, 1980, p. 56.

The emphasis and high investment in Tertiary Health Care is not a phenomenon confined to Barbados. Although there has been much rhetoric about Health For All by the Year 2000, one does not see a major change underway in most developing countries (or some developed countries, for that matter). There is also major expenditure on tertiary care institutions for most. One reason cited for this was that:

> Those who control health and budgets in developing countries are far too often urban-based and middle-class oriented and favour an allocation of health resources that replicates the hospital-based care patterns and the highly technical medical education of industrialized countries. Moreover, since political lead-

ers in developing countries ordinarily rely for health policy advice on doctors who are highly trained in modern clinical medicine, this misappropriation often tends to be given professional credibility.[62]

This observation is certainly true for Barbados where the majority of health care practitioners are in fact middle class, have offices that are urban-based or within close proximity of the urban population, and are medically focused.

Health Policy and Administration

The BLP's policy in relation to health was outlined in their 1979 to 1983 Development Plan:

> The government of Barbados strongly supports the views that health is a fundamental human right and that the attainment of the highest level of health is a most important social goal, whose realization requires the action of many other social and economic sectors in addition to the health sector. Further, the government views health services as an essential component of the socio-economic system and considers that the services should be targeted to protect and improve the health of every individual as well as the entire community.[63]

However despite this mandate, the existing private/public dichotomy produces (as noted in the same document) a "disparity" in health care delivery:

> This disparity is apparently due to the fact that the health care services, as they relate to the individual care, are delivered by both private and public providers...private doctors....(and) public medical services.... Thus, although it may be argued that anyone in Barbados can receive free medical care at the acute general hospital or the clinics, one is forced to concede that in practice, especially in primary care, immediate access to these services is not readily available to all health consumers.[64]

The BLP government in their Development Plan of 1979 to 1983 acknowledged that economic development, defined in terms of increase in per capita income, was not a measure indicating that health care services were reaching vulnerable groups. The government admitted to inequities and inefficiencies within the administration and delivery of health services and the prime minister, Tom Adams, pointed out that "access to high quality services in the present health care system is based on financial criteria rather than on the most efficient and effective way of providing health care to consumers."[65] Adams further decribed the present health services offered as "pauper medicine," noting that a strategy was needed to reach those who might have been by-passed by economic growth and are worst affected by inflationary trends.

The Development Plan conclusively declared that these neglected areas of the health care system could only be addressed by a change in policy direction towards the provision of Primary Health Care.

> It is obvious that such an approach would also cost less since it is much more expensive to treat illness after it occurs than if it is prevented in the first place. It is apparent that if we primarily rely upon treating illnesses to maintain the population's health, the costs will become so great that the public will not be able to maintain present health care standards.[66]

The BLP seemed to be aware of the political and ideological aspects that accompanied its policy in a class-based society, and acknowledged that the changes envisaged to make "Health for All" a reality required "unequivocal" commitment from the entire government and not just the Ministry of Health or the health sector.

> the introduction or strengthening of the development process needed to attain health for all will require unequal political commitment (emphasis added) to bring about reforms that are essential to convert this goal into reality. This will be set in motion by political decisions taken by the Government as a whole, and permeating all sectors at all levels throughout the country.[67]

The government was also cognizant that measures were needed to ensure community participation and to promote self-care and responsibility among individuals and communities, and that these measures were a "social, economic and technical necessity."[68]

NHS: The BLP's Proposal

A National Health Service (NHS) system was proposed as early as 1976 in the BLP's Manifesto. According to the Barbadian government, the decision to implement the NHS system and establish the polyclinics was in keeping with its goal of decentralization and integration of services at the community level and to ensure "that every person has access to all facets of the country's health services and that the ability to pay for services at the time of delivery will not be a determining factor."[69] It was projected that, through the introduction of a series of services over a period of time, the system would be implemented by 1981. The operational guidelines for NHS were as follows:[70]

- the National Health Service will operate within the framework of the present National Insurance Scheme;
- each citizen will be assigned to the doctor of his or her choice;
- each National Health Service Medical Practitioner will have and maintain a register or panel of patients;
- patients will not pay fees to the doctor;
- doctors will be remunerated on a "capitation basis," i.e., a fixed sum per year for each registered patient; and
- the prices of drugs prescribed by doctors to patients within the health service will be reduced and standardized.

The Barbados Drug Service was the first aspect program of the NHS to be implemented. Established in 1980, its mandate was to develop mechanisms for the containment, and where possible the reduction, of the cost of drugs to the consumer. A Special Benefit Service was started in 1981 and provided drugs free or at a subsidized cost to all residents 65 years of age and over; to children under 6 years of age; and to persons who required drugs for the treatment of hypertension, diabetes and/or cancer.

The next phase would have been the implementation of the General Practitioner Service within the framework of the polyclinics; this was to encourage the rationalization of the delivery of health care at the primary, secondary and tertiary levels and to promote a system based on health needs.[35] Persons 65 years and over were classified as Group A patients and were to be registered with a panel general practitioner who would deliver services at their private practices or at the polyclinics (which were expected to function as an integral component of the NHS). In relation to the general practitioner service within the NHS, a former Minister of health during the BLP administration pointed out that:

> the plan was to have doctors working in the polyclinics in order to provide care to people who could not afford to go to a private doctor. Prior to the development of the polyclinics concept, the health centres mainly provided Maternal and Child Health Services and we had hoped to expand that service to include a walk-in clinic with services for senior citizens and other special clinics. We had intended to staff the polyclinics with General Practitioners who would work on a rota system. We had decided to put the GPs on a 'per capita' rather than a "fee for service" but they didn't like the idea. We were mainly looking at two categories of doctors, young doctors who needed to start and build a practice and older ones who wanted to scale down their practice as they approached retirement. We had developed an attractive benefit package to the service but that did not work out. What I felt needed to be negotiated was the position of the specialists. We wanted them to behave as specialists and to discontinue their role of being both GPs and specialists.... as we were not going to be paying them for GP services.[72]

The Minister of Health in his defense of the NHS Bill stated in the senate that:

> The estimated expenditure per annum during the GP services for the Elderly Phase was $3.9 million. The total remuneration (including expenses) to be paid to the 60 doctors who will provide the services will range from $2.9 million to $3.1 million or approximately

76% to 80% of the total expenditure. In the final phase the GP services were to be made available to all residents at a projected total annual cost of $21.4 million with a maximum of 100 doctors inclusive of doctors expenses. The total remuneration to be paid to the doctors was between 92% and 95 % of the total expenditure.[73]

With these calculations, the government argued that the proposed NHS was more cost-effective and would save monies that were presently being spent on the fragmented services of the district out-patient clinics (which would be abolished); on the walk-in clinics of the Queen Elizabeth Hospital and the Polyclinics; as well as on the District Medical Officers since these posts will be abolished when the National Health Service Board's services are fully established (within 6 months of the introduction of the GP Service for the elderly).[74]

NHS: Implementation Problems

The NHS plan was, however, strongly opposed by the Barbados Association of Medical Practitioners (BAMP) from the onset. Efforts to make the polyclinics more functional and to get general practitioners into the communities fell short. In fact, the NHS was never fully implemented and by 1986 was abandoned.

BAMP felt the "system advocated will do the services of this country more harm than good. The resources of physicians are not yet available. If implemented at this time it will not improve the standard of care, rather we envisage a spread of perfunctory care, because of the heavy loading factor."[75] Two BAMP officials who were involved in different aspects of the NHS negotiations (with the government), stated that "there were several reasons why the doctors were unhappy with the BLP administration."[76] According to a BAMP representative, some of the Association's concerns were:[77]

1. The inefficiencies of the NHS in Britain. Although services were initially free, gradually people were paying more and more for care.
2. The lower pay would have demotivated panel general practitioners to the point where their performance was mechan-

ical consisting of just writing prescriptions and getting through numbers because they were covered by insurance. This, they claimed, was the situation in Britain.

3. The government was trying to exert too much control. For example, private practitioners would be required to maintain a register of patients. This guideline, which was the first ever of its kind in the history of medical care in Barbados, would have succeeded in making private practitioners as accountable as their counterparts working in the public sector. Another sore point articulated by the doctors was "they were being asked to be on call and to work longer hours. For in order for the polyclinic concept to work the clinic would have had to remain open for 18 hours a day until 7:00-8:00 at night instead of closing at 4:00 p.m. as they now do." In addition the service had promised to provide medical coverage on a twenty-four hour basis.

4. Negotiations were hampered by the numerous changes in Ministers of Health, at least five during the negotiation period including Tom Adams (then prime minister).

5. If Tom Adams, who was anti-Grenada, succeeded in getting the St. George's Medical School relocated to Barbados this would infringe on the current medical program operating at UWI.

Another area of disagreement between BAMP and the government was that the proposed plans for the introduction of the NHS were made without prior consultation with the Association.[78] The BLP had commissioned the Kaiser Foundation International, a non-profit U.S. based organization to study the feasibility of the NHS. (Funding for the study was provided by the Inter-American Development Bank (IADB) under an agreement with the government of Barbados) The Kaiser Foundation failed to consult with BAMP during the period of time it had been operating in Barbados. One of the BAMP officials also noted that the government had not addressed several issues of importance to the Association, including remuneration and terms of service. On the issue of pay, the following defence was given:

> I think that certainly it is wrong to say that a doctor in private practice should not be interested in money. I do think that patient care is exceedingly important

but if you are looking at a situation where you are asking a doctor providing a service not to make a profit but to take a loss then what is the benefit to anyone. What will happen under those circumstances is that either no doctors will participate or if they do participate then economic constraints will impact negatively against the patients if doctors tried to save cost simply to make ends meet and not to make a loss. So I don't think that patients would have benefited from that kind of service at all.[79]

BAMP claimed that, before the BLP proposed the NHS in their 1976 Party Manifesto, they had already discussed a service in which the most high risk and deserving people would be assured high quality care at reasonable costs to the tax payers. The retention of the fee-for-service represented a fundamental difference between the BLP's NHS policy and BAMP's strategic views.

Government policy is based on what they perceive as the "social and economic" wishes of *all* Barbadians, their desire to have a doctor of their choice, whom they will not have to pay at the time of consultation. BAMP has never been opposed to the NHS except to warn government that this system had proved very expensive in Britain, Europe and Canada where it was in operation. It must also be stated that the proposed NHS is not needed to improve the health status of Barbadians. In the past 30 years our health indices in the form of infant mortality rates, birth rates and life expectancy have improved, and demonstrate unequivocally that Barbadians are among the healthier in the world. There is no study nor any authority on health care that can recommend that the proposed NHS will further improve the health status of Barbadians. BAMP's policy would have sought to direct care to the most needy groups in the society, the elderly, those unfortunate people who suffer chronic diseases and need continuous care for the rest of their lives, the under 6 years old etc. We feel that this more prudent and effective use of costly health services will help to further improve the health status of the people.[80]

However a senior International Health Official disagreed with BAMP's explanation claiming that it was "too simplistic and it is more than it appeared to be," and instead stated that:

> the reason goes back to the difficulty of transferring power, putting power in people, it is a general problem, and if we take the whole Primary Care Approach, every single time when government say they have Primary Health Care everybody pays the rhetoric to it, very few however have empowered the people and have had genuine social participation because that is seen as threatening not only for the politicians but the professionals. So people come to the Polyclinics but then back off when it comes to the social participation and the empowerment of people.[81]

This issue of "transferring power" and empowering consumers is an important one that will be revisited throughout the study, particularly in review of the health systems from the women's perspective.

Human Resource Planning

Official sources differ on the number of doctors available in Barbados. 1980 figures show a difference ranging from 1:2000 to 1:2700 and as high as 1:5000.[82] Dann argued that the "anomalies in the official statistics, confusion over the extent of existing manpower may be indicative of lack of efficiency in the service and poor communication between the authorities and medical personnel. (Table 6.3 shows the breakdown of doctors, nurses, and other health care personnel)

The major training institution of choice for Caribbean doctors is still the University of the West Indies, Medical School. The majority of doctors however continue to focus in traditional and more prestigious areas of the medical profession. Although postgraduate training in the area of Public Health is available not many doctors specialize in this area. Advanced training and continuing medical education takes place locally, regionally and internationally.

Training for nursing staff was considered a priority. Nurses either were trained locally or sought further education at "foreign" institutions. During 1981, a mental health component was added to the basic nursing programme at the Barbados Community College so that "nurses graduating in the new system will be able to perform either in a general or a mental hospital"; seventy-eight nurses were expected to benefit from this training.[83] Despite these efforts to broaden the scope of opportunities available to nurses, the number of nursing personnel remained relatively the same from 1979 to 1982 with only slight fluctuations from year to year; 1982 to 1983 experienced a more noticeable drop from 546 to 519.[84]

In 1983, a Health Education Unit was established on a trial basis "in an effort to correct the fragmentary health education services."[85] A Health Education Officer was assigned as the Coordinator of the Unit which included the Public Health Educator of the Animal and Human Health Programs, the Research Officer of the Project Design and Implementation Unit, and four Family Life Educators based at polyclinics. Although the officers were assigned to the unit, they did not actually work out of the unit but remained in their present locations and were accountable not to the Health Education Coordinator, but to their immediate supervisors for any "specific assignments" carried out. The Health Educators proved to be ineffective; inadequately trained or equipped to perform their tasks; the programmes they delivered were inefficient. A six-month project review revealed that the "arrangement was unsatisfactory and the recommendation made sometime previously for a separate Health Education Division was again suggested."[86] ("The development of an effective Health Education Unit did not materialise" as of 1988.[87])

SUMMARY

Although Barbados modified and made some changes to its economic structure, it nevertheless continued to function as a neocolonial state dominated by international capital.[36] Despite the fact that the state introduced a number of Welfare programs for the poor and commissioned a major study on women, events show that neither group was adequately served. In particular working-class women experienced high unemployment, unequal access to training in non-traditional areas, and pay inequity; and women in general continue to be under-represented at the various strategic decision-making levels of the State machinery. In general the Barbadian health system was skewed towards curative care rather than health education and preventative services (PHC). Even the NHS concept, which represented a significant attempt to address the identified "inequities" within the system, was merely an extension of a medical model, ill equipped to address Primary Health Care issues as elucidated in the Alma Ata Declaration. How these systemic issues of inequities and resource imbalance affected the health of women and the ability of the government to address their health needs will be investigated through interviews with provider, administrators and consumers.

Table 6.3
Manpower (Barbados):
Health Personnel with Population Ratio 1979–1983

Category	1980 Total	# Persons To Each	1981 Total	# Persons To Each	1982 Total	# Persons To Each	1983 Total	#Persons To Each
Hospital Admins.	6	41, 500	6	41,567	6	41,732	6	41,873
Doctors	212	1,200	218	1,144	221	1,133	213	1,180
Nurses & Nurse/ midwives	571	440	534	467	546	459	519	484
Public Health Nurses	44	5,700	49	5,090	46	5,443	55	4,568
Psychiatric nurses	145	1,700	164	1,521	155	1,615	170	1,478
Midwives	30	8,300	37	6,741	36	6,741	40	6,281
Nursing) Assistants (trained & untrained)	402	3,410	405	3,327	400	3,407	390	3,717
Radiographers, Laboratory technicians/	260	21, 300	274	21,450	273	21,651	174	21,196

Table 6.3 Cont'd

Manpower (Barbados):

Category	1980 Total	# Persons To Each	1981 Total	# Persons To Each	1982 Total	# Persons To Each	1983 Total	#Persons To Each
technicians & Dispensers Physiotherapists, Occupational therapists (OT) & OT assistants	18	287,800	17	293,978	18	153,017	18	188,430
Public health inspectors (qualified & unqualified)	100	15,100	102	20,648	95	30,933	97	25,761
Sanitary Engineers & Public Health engineering assist.	10	155,600	12	94,525	11	114,763	10	157,025
Dentists & Dental assist.	37	32,200	38	32,910	42	29,212	38	29,376

Source: Annual Report of the Chief Medical Officer of Health, 1983 Ministry of Health, Barbados, pp. 50-52.

Notes

1. Hilary Beckles. *A History of Barbados: from Amerindian Settlement to Nation-state*: Cambridge University Press, 1990:170.
2. Ibid.
3. Ibid.:171.
4. Ibid.:17.
5. Ibid.:176.
6. Ibid.
7. Gordon K. Lewis *The Growth of the Modern West Indies*: Monthly Review Press, 1968:192.
8. Ibid.
9. Ibid.:242.
10. Ibid. see also Beckles, 1990.

11. "Errol Walton Barrow - Patriot, Friend of the Working People and Outstanding Politician"; A tribute by Michael Manley in Speeches by Errol Barrow (ed.), Yusif Haniff: 1987:13 Hansib Publishing Limited, 1987:13.
12. Ibid.:14.
13. Carl Stone. *Power in the Caribbean Basin: A Comparative Study of Political Economy* Inter-American Politics Series, 1986:129 see also Beckles, 1990.
14. Hilary Beckles. (1) (990):203.
15. Ibid.:204; see also Stone, 1986; Thomas, 1988
16. Ibid.:205, see also Thomas, 1988
17. Member countries included Dominica, St Lucia, Jamaica, St. Vincent, and Barbados. Thomas, 1988, p.343.
18. Fitzroy Ambursley and James Dunkerley. Grenada Whose Freedom? London: Latin American Bureau, 1984:105.
19. Hilary Beckles (1990): 205.
20. Jamaica and Guyana officially recognized Grenada, See LeRoy Taylor, *Economic Adjustments and Health Care Financing in the Caribbean,* Institute of Social and Economic Research, University of the West Indies, Mona Jamaica, 1990.
21. David Renwick and David Jessop, "Grenada Special: Grenada Revolution: A Major Setback for Regional Unity 1979" News Analysis, 1979 :4.
22. Clive Thomas. *The Poor and the Powerless: Economic Policy and Change in the Caribbean* Latin American Bureau, 1988:273.
23. Ibid. (quoting Jainarain): 268-269.
24. Ibid.:269.
25. Ibid.:276; Gairy S Fields, *Growth, Employment, Inequality and Poverty in Trinidad, Barbados and Jamaica*: Department of Economics, Cornell University, Working Paper 41. December, 1981.
26. Barbados Development Plan 1979 to 1983, Chapter 1
27. Tom Adams, the Prime Minister and Minister of Finance and Planning, 1978 Budget Speech: Barbados Development Plan 1979-1983, Chapter 1.
28. Ibid.
29. Gairy Fields (1981):4-8.
30. It is impossible to directly determine how income was distributed since no data changes in equality and poverty were noted during this time frame See Fields, 1981.
31. The Barbados Development Bank's Annual Report 1979-80, p25
32. Y Haniff, "Emergency Powers, Now in Barbados" (Caribbean Contact 1982).
33. Ibid.
34. Ibid.

35. Adams, J.M.G, Prime Minister and Minster of Finance and Planning, Barbados Financial Statement and Budgetary Proposal: Wednesday, April 27, 1983:3.
36. Ibid.1983:5.
37. Ibid.
38. Hilary Beckles (1990):205.
39. Hughes, 1978:4.
40. Norma Forde. "The Report of the National Commision on the Status of Women :What Has Been Done.": 1979.
41. Where Are we Now? An Assessment of the Status of Women in Barbados: Bureau of Women's Affairs, Ministry of Labour and Community Development, 1983:31.
42. House of Assembly Debates (Official Report, Second Session 1976 to 1981):1.
43. Norma Forde (1979):22-23.
44. Scarlette L. Gillings. "Review of the Barbados Women's Bureau" Port of Spain, Trinidad: Study prepared for the ILO subregional Office, Oct., 1987:7.
45. Ibid.
46. Ibid.:8.
47. Ibid.
48. Ibid.:12
49. Ibid.:14
50. Medical Termination of Pregnancy Act (1983 to 1984):2.
51. Varda Burstyn. "Masculine dominance and the State." Varda Burstyn and Dorothy Smith. *Women, Class and the State:* Garamond Press, 1985:72.
52. Norma Forde (1983):22.
53. Graham Dann. *The Quality of Life in Barbados.*: Macmillan Caribbean, 1984: 149.
54. Ibid.:147.
55. Medical Officer of Health Report, Ministry of Health, 1984.
56. Medical Officers Report (1983):11.
57. Barbados Development Plan (1979 to 1983):138.
58. Leroy Taylor (1988):7.
59. Graham Dann (1984).
60. Barbados Development Plan (1979 to 1983):140.
61. Ibid.:147.
62. Jacques Vallen & Alan D. Lorez (eds.) *Health Policy, social Policy and Mortality Prospects:* International Union of Scientific Study of Population, 1985: 501.
63. Barbados Development (1979 to 1983):137.
64. Ibid.:138.
65. Ibid.
66. Ibid.:137.

67. Ibid.:138.
68. Ibid.:139.
69. Ibid.
70. Health Service Development Plan 1983 to 1987 (Ministry of Health, Barbados, 1984).
71. Ibid.:1.
72. Interview, September 1992.
73. O'Brien Trotman. "Statement delivered by the Minister of Health Re the NHS bill at the Twelfth Meeting of the Senate." : Wed 20th June, 1984:5.
74. Trotman (1984):5.
75. BAMP Discussion Paper on the proposed NHS (1979): 15.
76. Ibid.
77. Interview, September 1992.
78. See BAMP Discussion Paper (1979).
79. Interview, November 1992.
80. Interview, September 1992.
81. Interview, September 1992.
82. Graham Dann (1985):150.
83. Annual Report of the Chief Medical Officer of Health (1983): 55.
84. Ibid.:52.
85. Ibid.:53.
86. Ibid.
87. See Development Plan Ministry of Health (1988 to 1993):5.
88. See Carl Stone, Clive Thomas, 1988; Gordon Lewis 1983; and others.

CHAPTER 7

GRENADA

THE POLITICAL SITUATION

Prior to 1979

Grenada, a British colony from 1877 to 1967, was unique in that it escaped the labour unrest which occurred throughout the region during 1937 to 1938. Socio-economic conditions were, however, no different; the late 1940s and the 1950s were marred by low wages, harsh working environments, social discrimination and political disenfranchisement. These conditions forced the Grenadian people to organize themselves and push for change. In 1951, full adult suffrage was attained and the social uprisings occurring at the time brought Eric Matthew Gairy and the Grenada United Labour Party (GULP) into prominence. Gairy, who had first achieved power as a union leader in 1950, became an Official Representative under Her Majesty's Government in 1957 and Grenada's first native Prime Minister in 1973.[1] Known as "Uncle Gairy," he (and his administration) strongly identified with the working class, gaining most of their support from the rural population. His popularity among the working poor during the 1950s, can be likened to that of another

popular Caribbean leader, Errol Barrow, (known as the "Dipper")
of Barbados.

In 1967, Grenada became an Associated State of Britain; this
meant that Grenada had full autonomy in domestic affairs, but
Britain retained responsibility for defence and external affairs.[2]
During GULP's term of office from 1967 to 1979, Gairy
"became increasingly anti-working-class"[3] and began using several harsh measures to ensure loyalty, especially that of the public servants; the fear of victimization and financial insecurity kept
people from taking opposition. Similarly, Gairy began to control
businesses by granting favourable licence privileges to those who
supported him. The young working-class people, however, unlike
their parents, did not support Gairy. In fact,

> the mere mention of Gairy's name among the 15-30
> age group was sufficient to evoke revulsion and even
> hostility. The young had nothing to remember him
> for; some of their parents (especially the poor) who
> lived through and benefited from the 1951 "social
> revolution" idolized him, and his popularity among
> them fed upon his first impression. But the young,
> who lived through the 1970s, could remember only
> inflation, unemployment and acts of brutality, some-
> times sporadic, sometimes widespread. Gairy's name
> became anathema to the young; in politics he was
> their bete noire.[4]

The growing dissatisfaction with Gairy's undemocratic tendencies
led youth, women, intellectuals and members of the working-class
to organize and form groups in protest.

The Formation of the NJM

The New Jewel Movement (NJM), formed in 1973, was one of
the organizations that grew out of the discontent with GULP and
was successful in attracting a large segment of the youthful population who were influenced by the American Black Power Movement of the 1960s and similar activities in socialist States such
as Tanzania.[5] The NJM linked with other anti-Gairy opposition
groups to form the "Committee of Twenty-two" (a strong coali-

tion of union leaders, teachers, professionals and business people) whose objectives of restoring democratic liberties coincided with the NJM Party's 1973 Manifesto (Power to the People) which supported and promoted:

> a whole range of far-reaching programmes: agricultural reform, agro-industries, free secondary education, curriculum reform and freedom schools, a national health insurance scheme and preventive medicine campaigns, social planning, new tourism, the nationalization of banks, the phasing-out of foreign insurance companies and the establishment of a government-owned National Insurance Company....The Manifesto also called for an end to party politics and the institution of People's Assemblies as the political structure that would ensure participatory democracy and the permanent involvement of all the people in decision-making.[6]

The NJM immediately began to organize its followers into "cells at their places of work or residence and to mobilize them for political action"[7] around independence, the main issue on the Party's agenda. The NJM did not envisage the traditional form of independence (the so called flag raising ceremony) but instead "demanded independence projects not celebrations, it demanded negotiations with the British for partial reparation for wealth exported to them from Grenada during three centuries or so of British rule."[8] This 1973 period of intensive mobilization of the Grenadian peoples saw several members and supporters of the NJM were beaten, maimed and killed by the State security forces.[9] The "Committee of Twenty-two," however, continued to receive the support of the Grenadian people and thus presented a new challenge to the State. They were able to sustain an island-wide strike from January-March 1974, but were unsuccessful in toppling the Gairy regime as anticipated.

Despite the continued political unrest and the failing popularity of Gairy and the GULP government locally and regionally, the British government nevertheless granted Grenada independence under the leadership of Eric Gairy on February 7, 1974. With the country's new independent status, Gairy now had official state powers which allowed him to run the island as he saw fit. In addition to his national power, Gairy also gained entry into the United Nations and the Organization of American States (OAS). At these fora, the new Prime Minister denounced his opponents as communists and called for concerted action to be taken against the "left" throughout the Caribbean. The capability of the army and other security forces were also strengthened through military aid and training in Chile from the Pinochet dictatorship,[10] and close links were established with the authoritarian regime of Park Chun Hee in South Korea.[11]

Stone, a Caribbean intellectual who supported Bishop's "leftist populist-statist regime," argued that although Eric Gairy had ruled under a "Westminster-style parliamentary democracy," he had nonetheless made the

> democratic-pluralist state system into an authoritarian regime between Independence in 1974 and 1979. Elections were rigged, power was abused and opposition groups and politicians were subjected to violence.[12]

The Building of the NJM

The NJM, during its first year, had gained experience in mobilizing the Grenadian people for political action and continued to strengthen its position through educational and organizational work. The party's newspaper, *The New Jewel,* increased its circulation to 10,000 copies from a few hundred.[13] The NJM established local groups in almost every village and held frequent meetings despite continued harassment by Gairy's supporters. By 1976, the NJM had succeeded in securing and broadening its popular support and was able to gain the support of a wide cross-section of the Grenadian population. However, although their meetings received wide public support, the party itself did not increase in membership. This may be attributed to the fact that up to this point "the NJM was more a movement than a party for, although it was fighting on a clear set of issues, it lacked a strategic programme and cohesive internal organization."[14] This sense of direction and cohesiveness was said to have been achieved only with Bernard Coard's return to Grenada in 1976. Coard, a Marxist economist and educator, was "a committed proponent of the 'non-capitalist path of development' projected by the Soviet Union and Cuba for Third World Countries; and played a leading role in drawing the party towards official communism."[15] Although NJM's change in the ideology to a Marxist-Leninist position was not officially made, several progressive movements and Marxist groups within and outside the Caribbean began to identify with the party. Many of the leaders of these groups had lost respect for Gairy, but nevertheless remained cautious about their total acceptance of NJM, the new radicalism that was gaining strength.

The development of the NJM took place at two levels; while they continued to participate in the political activities of the "undemocratic state," they also proceeded to build a small core of "socialists cadres" who participated in a small study group known as the Organization of Revolutionary Education and Liberation (OREL). This group, which had Marxist-Leninist tendencies, "was to gain increasing influence"[16] over the NJM. During the 1979 elections, the NJM also formed an alliance with other anti-Gairy parties to contest the up-coming elections.

1979 to 1983

The alliance won 48 percent of the votes and six seats in the chamber; the NJM took three seats and Maurice Bishop became leader of the opposition.[17] This was a great feat since the opposition fought the election campaign under heavy government pressure and harassment from the Mongoose Gang who actively broke up their meetings. The GULP won the elections and returned to power in 1979 with nine seats; however, Gairy's "legitimacy had been substantially eroded."[18]

Despite the presence of a legitimate opposition force, Gairy continued his despotic rule and hardened his position against elected members by enforcing statutes which had been introduced earlier, such as the Firearms Act (1968), which rescinded all firearms permits to members of the opposition; the Public Order Act (1974), which permitted the use of loudspeakers by the police only; the Newspaper Act (1975), which required a deposit of nearly US $9,000 to be made to the State before publication was allowed; and the Essential Services and Port Authority Acts, which prohibited strikes of any kind. On the personal front Gairy continued to accumulate property for himself, disburse official funds, force sexual favours from women in the civil service, and indulge his fascination with the supernatural.[19] It was precisely because of Gairy's unpredictable modus operandi that the NJM began to gain more support from state employees, among them the police and sectors of the army. The contacts in the security forces later proved to be vital to the NJM in their efforts to seize power, and "it was through them that arms were acquired and the rudiments of the party's People's Revolutionary Army (PRA) was established."[20]

The Revolution

Through their contacts in the army, the leadership of the NJM learned of GULP's plans to arrest and eliminate them. Following the departure of Prime Minister Gairy from the island on Monday, March 12, 1979, the party decided to take control of the country. Early on the morning of March 13, about 40 members of the NJM took control of the True Blue Army barracks and began to mobilize the population by radio. According to Jules,

> the people rallied to the NJM, taking to the streets and providing whatever support was needed to consolidate the overthrow of the regime. Women, workers and unemployed youth played a prominent role in the insurrection.[21]

The entire operation, according to Ambursley & Dunkerley, took only 12 hours with no concerted resistance and only three deaths[22]; and thus Grenada, according to Stone,

> abandoned democratic pluralism thereby indicating a major shift away from the inherited tradition of politics.... The overriding factor which contributed to the change in style of government was the abuse of power by the political executive.[23]

For the people of Grenada there was a sense of relief at Gairy's demise and cause for much celebration; for the NJM, taking over the State was a huge responsibility.

The People's Revolutionary Government

The NJM, on taking power, assumed the name of the People's Revolutionary Government (PRG); the new government was made up of trade union leaders, independent professionals and members of the business class. The core members, who also occupied positions in the Peoples' Revolutionary Army (PRA), formed the Central Committee and were responsible for monitoring a number of Party subcommittees. The two most powerful of which were the executive bodies, the Organizing Committee (OC) and the Political Bureau (PB). Ambursley & Dunkerley argued that although

> the political bureau, a sub-committee of the Central Committee, was the body responsible for the development of overall policy; it was the PRG which was vested with legislative and executive powers and with which Grenadians most strongly identified themselves.[24]

This division of power was however merely organizational since real power was not controlled totally by the PRG (which represented the state) but by the Central Committee of the Party which remained a tight top-down structure with a membership of approximately 300 persons. This hegemony of party over state bore close resemblance to what had occurred in Guyana where the paramountcy of the ruling party, the Peoples National Congress (PNC), took precedence over the State in all matters. Although, the division in power and control between the party and the State seemed uneven and the structure distinctly hierarchical, Jules argued that "the NJM employed a wide variety of approaches and methods of party organization in relation to the state and mass organizations."[25]

This ability of the NJM to ensure that consensus was maintained within its ranks was attributed largely to Bishop's democratic form of leadership and popularity among the masses. Ambursley & Dunkerley noted that although

> Bishop was a convinced radical and although he was from the start the figurehead of the Grenadian revolution, he always presided over a government that was organised along collective lines.[26]

(Several writers and political commentators have claimed that Bernard Coard, deputy prime minister at the time, was the "real leader" of the revolution.[27])

One of the first acts of the revolution was the suspension of the independence constitution. This was done with assurances to return constitutional rule, including free elections and religious and political opinions.[28] However since this was not a collective view within the NJM, the PRG was forced not to take any steps that would return Grenada to a "Westminster" style constitutional rule and elections.

One of the most celebrated aspects of the revolution was the

> impulse which it gave to the self-organization of society at large. As a result of legislation and initiatives made by the NJM there was a prodigious growth in the strength of the popularity of the mass organizations-the National Women's Organization (NWO); the National Youth Organization (NYO); the People's Revolutionary Militia; the National School Students' Council and Pioneers.[29]

As early as 1974, the NJM had established and built links with various women's groups, youths groups and other associations so that by 1978 there was a network of party support groups in each parish which formed the nucleus of the revolution. After the revolution, these parish councils continued to function as forums for open dialogue between the leadership and the people. Ambursley & Dunkerley noted that because the groups mushroomed so quickly a decision was made to break down each of the 6 parishes into 36 zones which were representative of the population. The National Women's Organization (NWO) and National Youth Organization (NYO), the militia, the Productive Farmers' Union and others[30] worked along with the zonal councils so that issues concerning the various sectors or regions were discussed at various monthly forums. The leadership of the NJM, ministers of government, senior government officials and personnel of government departments participated in these meetings to give an account of their work, explain new programs and respond to questions and criticisms. This new form of "open government" practiced by the PRG during the early days ensured that the state was accountable to the people. All subsequent major pieces of legislation passed were discussed in meetings and mass organizations, the process of consultation being built into the PRG's system of popular power. In 1982, this system was widened to include the presentation of the budget to the people for their criticisms, suggestions and recommendations.

This format of governance marked a new era of policy development in Grenada and the rest of the English-speaking Caribbean, a model that emphasized the involvement and participation of ordinary Grenadians. Although the PRG government was not strictly "constitutional" it represented a more participatory approach than any of the other Caribbean governments in the English-speaking Caribbean. The Westminister model used by the others lacked this ongoing public participation and instead, they were constructed around a formal apparatus in which elections took place every few years. Public involvement was limited to these times. The system of popular consultation and debate reflected the PRG's success in "establishing itself as the norm rather than an exciting aberration"[31] and as such, Maurice Bishop proposed to make the local councils part of the government machinery.

Under the PRG administration, eight new trade unions were formed. Most of them led by NJM members, and several laws were introduced including the People's Law No. 29 of 1979 which stipulated that workers were free to join a union of their collective preference, determined by a secret ballot of at least 50 percent of the workers in each workplace. This new decree resulted in an average of 70-80 percent of all workers on the island being unionized.[32] The reintroduction of these democratic measures allowed the government to maintain their programmes as well as their popularity during the severe economic crisis affecting the entire region. The new Grenadian state was said to be "moreover, signally devoid of corruption in distinction to almost every other contemporary government in the Caribbean".[33]

Jules, claimed that the PRG experienced increased pressures from the newly elected Reagan administration from 1980 on:

> the revolution was faced with unrelenting effects of US hostility and opposition in international financial organization.... In March 1981 it succeeded in blocking a US$6.3 million capital project development loan and

US$3 million in concessionary assistance from the World Bank.[34]

This loan was to be used on capital projects in agriculture, agro-industry, tourism and housing. In July 1981, the US Government failed in an attempt to exclude Grenada from accessing funds from the Caribbean Development Bank (CDB), a regional agency, but the accumulation of such pressures led to cash flow problems and pushed the PRG government into consolidating its financial resources to make sure that its principal economic priority, the completion of the international airport at Pointe Saline (to attract tourists), was met.

THE ECONOMIC SITUATION

Prior to 1979

The economy of Grenada, like those of other "small island" states in the Eastern Caribbean, constitutes a classic case of openness and foreign domination, features consistent with its long history of colonialism and the nature of its resource base in export agriculture and tourism.[35] The fragile nature of the economy and its external dependence were in a sense made complete by the historically volatile and declining terms of trade of agricultural products, along with the economic conditions prevailing in developed countries. During the period 1965 to 1970, under the Gairy administration, the Grenadian economy underwent significant structural changes. Agriculture, which had held a position of dominance, declined from 38.9 percent to 29.9 percent of the GDP, tourism increased from 3 percent to 5.2 percent (decreased in the 1973 to 1974 period) and manufacturing accounted for 5.2 percent; however the government bureaucracy, which was built on political patronage, increased from 13.4 percent to 23.2 percent of the GDP.[36] According to reports coming out of organizations such as the World Bank, GULP was refused several loans due to its "inadequate managing and accounting practices"[37] and "because of the incompetence and corruption"[38] of its leaders and administrators. Offers refused or rescinded included: a loan from the Caribbean Development Bank under the Small Industry Credit Scheme; $5.7 million from the European Development Bank; and

US$175,000 from the Organization of Petroleum Exporting Countries (OPEC).[39] During the last year of Gairy's rule, Grenada was behind in its constitutional levy payments and consequently almost lost its membership in the UN, UNESCO, WHO, the University of the West Indies and other organizations.[40] The combination of these economic and social disasters hastened the termination of Gairy's rule.

1979 to 1983

Jules argued that because the situation inherited from Gairy was so dismal in terms of the mismanagement of the economy and rising unemployment:

> [d]iversification was therefore used [by the PRG] as a strategy for overcoming some of the limitations posed by dependency and the international division of labour on the structural autonomy of the state and was associated with Grenada's active policy positions on South issues such as the International Economic Order and its vigorous participation in the Non-aligned Movement. One result of this approach was.... Increased food production together with the diversification of trade resulted in an increase in export earnings of fruit and vegetables from EC$ 1.5 million in 1981 to EC$ 4.5 million in 1982.[41]

The economic strategy pursued by the PRG was described as "a "mixed economy model" comprised of the state sector, the private sector and the co-operative sector,"[42] with the state sector as the major partner comprising about 30-40 percent of the economy. The ability of the PRG to attract outside funding "helped to greatly improve the island's infrastructure and establish a number of state enterprises"[43] and to stimulate and improve the overall economy. As a result, "capital spending increased from EC$8 million under Gairy in 1978, to EC$16 million in 1979, EC$39.9 million in 1980, EC$79.2 million in 1981 and EC$101.5 million in 1982."[44] Compared to the other "small islands" or LDCs, Grenada was now spending more on its economy. (See Table 7.1)

Table 7.1
Government Revenue and Expenditure, 1981 (US$ Millions)

Country	Revenue	Expenditure	Surplus/Deficit
Antigua & Barbuda*	45.2	34.5	+10.6
Barbados	173.9	230.8	-56.9
Belize (a)	23.5	25.1	-1.6
Dominica*	27.3	31.1	-3.8
Grenada*	22.3	49.9	-27.6
Guyana	375.6	460.5	-84.9
Jamaica	804.4	1,442.1	(b)-637.7
Monsterrat*	(c)5.6	8.0 (b)	-2.4 (b)
St. Christopher -Nevis*	24.9	27.9	-3.0
St. Vincent & the Grenadines*	24.4	27.1	-2.7
Trinidad & Tobago	2,962.7	2,781.2	+181.5

* LDC countries;
(a) Figures for 1977 only; (b) Estimate only; (c) Figures for 1979 only.
Source: Sinha, Dinesh, P. *Children of the Caribbean 1945 to 1984,* 1988, p. 53.

Despite the severe economic and social problems confronting the PRG, the shortage of skilled personnel, high import costs of equipment and other necessary amenities, lack of commitment shown by some government officials and support from some of its CARICOM partners,

> the state was able to achieve significant gains through its mass mobilization strategies, its ability to fuse economic development objectives and geo-political strategic interests into an aggressive foreign policy, and prudent economic management initiatives.[45]

Most of the internally- and externally-raised funds were allocated to the construction of the airport which was seen as crucial to the economic development of the country's tourism and agricultural industries and became a national project. Substantial investments were also made in the tourism sector which suffered a loss in 1982 as a result of the international recession and negative reports made by the US media about Grenada. In early 1983, the government purchased the Holiday Inn hotel and "hired a private company to manage it."[46] By the end of 1983 the Minister of Tourism reported that visitors to the island had increased significantly.

The PRG was able to obtain a loan of US$2 million from the Caribbean Development Bank (CDB) to improve the State farms and to build three new agricultural training schools to "train youths in modern methods of farming";[47] this boosted the agricultural sector which was previously bankrupt. The PRG also initiated several agro-industrial enterprises and several products (e.g. saltfish, smoked herring, nutmeg jellies, and a variety of local fruit juices) were developed locally.[48] In addition to the State's intervention in agriculture, the PRG also set up the National Commercial Bank (NCB) and the Grenada Bank of Commerce. This decision was made after the Canadian Imperial Bank of Commerce and the Royal Bank of Canada decided to close their operations. In 1982, the NCB was reported as having deposits of more than EC$40 million and was lending more to agriculture and other productive areas of the economy than any other bank operating in Grenada.[49]

In 1979, the Grenadian economy began to grow and by 1983, the real GDP had risen by 5.5 per cent and the PRG was able "to reduce unemployment from the 50 per cent level that it was under Gairy to less than 14 per cent"; unemployment among youth (under 25 years of age) was particularly high, as much as 80 per cent.[50] The high level of unemployment:

> was responsible for continuous emigration and creating a population dependent upon remittances from relatives abroad; an economy based on the needs of Europe and the United States rather than that of the population; substandard housing and grossly inadequate health care; piped water and electricity available only to those able to pay; insufficient educational facilities, especially in rural areas producing high levels of illiteracy.[51]

One of the interesting features of the PRG administrative style was the strategy it used in developing its national budget development. Ambursley & Dunkerley noted that this was a rather elaborate exercise; the stages are outlined, as follows:

1. expenditure requests from all government departments were studied by the Ministry of Finance headed by Bernard Coard.
2. a preliminary draft was developed and submitted to the PRG cabinet for discussion.
3. the draft was presented by Ministry of Finance officials to mass organizations, trade unions, zonal and parish councils.
4. delegates from all of the mass organizations attended a national conference on the economy where they were given the task of critiquing the draft proposal.
5. the budget was then returned to the Ministry of Finance for final revisions, and then to cabinet for approval.
6. finally, a detailed report was presented to the people by the Ministry, this included explanations for the rejection of any recommendations that had been made.

Ambursley noted, however, that although the process involved a great deal of community involvement, the final decision-making power still rested with the PRG. Since, as will be discussed, the hierarchy of the PRG had only one woman, women's issues were not always considered a priority.

THE STATE AND WOMEN

Prior to 1979

The status of working class women in Grenada prior to the revolution was no different from that of women of the same class in other Caribbean islands of a similar colonial experience. For example, women's legal rights were unequal to those of men, and as late as

> 1971 a woman could not become a juror until the age of 30, while a man could do so at age 21; she had to obtain her husband's permission to take up permanent residence elsewhere; and according to the "Dumcasta Clause" in separation agreements, she could only receive alimony and maintenance for as long as she remained "chaste."[52]

Under the Gairy administration, sexual exploitation of women both by government officials and private employers was the norm. Unemployment for women was 69 percent and women performing manual labour were given far lower wages than their male counterparts even though they performed similar or comparable tasks.[53] This unfair wage practice was true not only in Grenada and Barbados as highlighted, but also in the rest of the region.[54]

1979 to 1983

Under the PRG, several changes were made in an attempt to address the gender inequities inherent in the system; these included the passing of legislation to abolish all forms of sexual discrimination. The PRG believed that women (and other sectors of the oppressed and exploited strata) should organize independently to represent their own interests and ensure that policies enacted by the State reflected their rights. Prime Minister Bishop reiterated this belief in the following statement:

> we feel that the most important beginning is when conscious, organized and united women themselves take the initiative in beginning to identify their problems.[55]

The Grenadian women were doing just this and had begun to organize themselves through the National Women's Organization (NWO), a grass-roots organization formed in 1978, and the Women's Desk, a ministerial body. The NWO was formed to "organize women in the whole process of the revolution" since formally they were not organized at the community level and lacked basic leadership skills. The organizational process involved training women not just as "students but as teachers so that they could go back into the community and train and organize"[56] ; it was designed to raise women's consciousness about the political situation of the country, as well as about themselves as women.

Although the NWO consisted of members of the former St. George's-based Women's Progressive Organization (WPO) and existed prior to the revolution, it did not develop into a mass organization until after the revolution. Comprised of 161 local groups from various towns and villages, the NWO by 1980 had become involved in different aspects of the national political, educational and health campaigns, from assisting the communities in drafting new "progressive legislation for equal rights" to women's participation in the People's Militia. The organization was also, in collaboration with the Women's Desk, instrumental in supporting women's rights to paid leave during pregnancy and in the Maternity Leave Law being passed in 1980, after intensive public debate with the PRG. Also high on the list of achievements were the development of pre-school and daycare centres, and a successful campaign for the removal of discrimination in pay and conditions.[57] Women not only participated in the organization and implementation of the literacy and adult education campaign but, as a group, benefited from the two programs.

The Women's Desk was also active in furthering the development of Grenadian women. According to Maurice Bishop, their function was to:[58]

1. Establish special commissions and participatory fora for review of the Laws "to ensure equality at least on the statute book";
2. Ensure adoption by government of the 1969 UN Resolution on the Discrimination of Women and other UN and international charters on the rights of women;
3. Ensure representation of women on all national bodies "so that they will have an input in every important area, so that they will be in a position to struggle at all times for the rights of women in our country";
4. Monitor progress on government declarations affecting women "to ensure that the law and its practice at all times approximate";
5. Become directly involved in the organization of women to promote their active presence in all revolutionary structures including their own autonomous structures;
6. Ensure participation of women in decision-making at all levels in government and society;
7. Monitor and get involved in the provision of social and economic services which would specifically benefit women (e.g. daycare centres, basic amenities in rural areas);
8. Participate in community development.

The Women's Desk changed to the Ministry of Women's Affairs in 1982 and was the only one of its kind in the region. (All other Caribbean governments have established Women's Desks and bureaus within a government ministry. Of course the uniqueness of the Grenadian situation was short lived for, after the tragic demise of the revolution in 1983, the status of the Women's Desk was reversed so that it was now in line with its regional partners.) The

PRG was, in effect, the only regional government administration which fully recognized the importance of women's affairs and accorded it full ministerial status. Joseph, a former leader of the National Women's Organization (NWO), stated that the PRG was committed to changing the status of women from the inception.

> The People's Revolutionary Government (PRG) of Grenada is firmly committed, not only to the principle of equal rights for women, but also to the active promotion of full and equal participation by women in all areas of the economy and society including their full participation and the ensuring of all social and legal rights and legal protection to women.[59]

Although the revolution provided women with opportunities at all levels of the society, in effect, "the revolution needed women to make their programs work."[60] This fact caused Porter to question whether the state gave women more freedom or whether it increased exploitation of women in the following statement:

> Both the Party and the Grenadian economy continued to rely on unpaid labour to support and build the social and economic base. Party supporters were encouraged to work overtime at their jobs and to undertake community work. Women in particular were encouraged to provide free baby-sitting for party members and contribute food and supplies for community and national events.[61]

These concerns were also expressed by senior women leaders who were critical of the chauvinistic actions and behaviour of certain male members within the Central Committee of the Party. A report submitted by the Chairperson of the Women's Committee, Phyllis Coard,[62] captured the lack of consideration for needs of female party members. Mrs. Coard argued that the insensitivity included: inappropriate meeting times, last minute summons to meetings, and the unavailability of child care facilities; the non-participation of (party) men in domestic work (while women members were expected to carry a full load of political responsibilities in addition to their domestic burdens); and the licentious behaviour of male party members. The report also asserted that it is time the party starts to formulate rules of personal behaviour on the man-woman question....and raise the ideological level of all party members on this matter. Too many party members do not see that the struggle for socialism includes the struggle to create socialist forms of relationships within our society.[63]

Joseph argued that women became very prominent in political positions in PRG administration rising from 2 in 1979 to 6 in 1981 (4 deputy ministers; 2 ambassadors). She also noted that senior civil servants increased from 2 in 1979 to 20. There were also appointments to several senior positions in public agencies and commissions statutory bodies.[64] Porter disagreed with Joseph claiming that not all of these women were in fact Grenadians[65]; however, Jules made a more substantial political observation when he stated that

[w]omen were increasingly involved at the policy making levels in the State apparatus but this representation was not reflected in the NJM itself. The membership of the highest party bodies, the Central Committee and the Political Bureau included only one woman (Phyllis Coard).[66]

This underrepresentation of women at the highest levels of the party meant that, while women (and working class women, in particular) were highly involved at the community level and gave support to the projects initiated by the government, input into policy decisions of the state was minimal. Issues critical to women's existence would, therefore, have been ignored; for example, neither the PRG nor the NWO considered the effect of this additional community responsibility on the health of women who were already overworked and had more or less full responsibility of caring for their children and families. This dual role, in fact, made the status of women more unfavourable and hindered the commitment made by the PRG to improve the "social, political and economic development of women."[67]

THE HEALTH CARE SYSTEM

Health Infrastructure

Prior to the revolution, Grenada's health care system was structurally similar to that of Barbados and most other colonial models, with both the private and public sectors providing primary, secondary and tertiary health care. Similarly, as in Barbados, most doctors and therefore services were located in the capital; there was an emphasis on curative measures; basic medical care was not available to all Grenadians; and the cost of private care was expensive and thus inaccessible to the working poor, the majority of whom were Black.

The Ministry of Health in November 1981 reported that they had inherited a poorly managed and maintained health system, including:[68]

1. Poor medical coverage of health care services; a particularly critical shortage of doctors and other trained personnel.
2. An acute shortage of existing services, supplies and equipment.
3. Low quality public health services as compared to the relative better quality of the private sector.
4. Very little preventative medicine or strictly remedial type services.
5. Problems in environmental health, shortage of trained public health inspectors and junior inspectors. Equipment for performing the functions of this department was not available in many instances.
6. Dilapidated and inadequate health care facilities and physical infrastructure in many institutions.
7. A large number of untrained health workers, causing a massive state of demoralization among health workers.

The working conditions of health personnel during the Gairy regime was summed up by a senior government official:

> The doctors who staffed the hospital were described as "tired and demoralized," because the demand at the hospital for care was far greater than its capacity to supply. It was also during this period that hospital nurses demonstrated against the worsening conditions of work, lack of transportation and uniforms. The nurses also complained of political interference in the recruitment of nurses.[69]

This was to change later, after the revolution and the adoption of primary health care. The PRG government began a process of identifying health needs and gaps in services and began to invest more in PHC initiatives. De Riggs, a former deputy minister of health stated that

> The PRG government had a deeper or more realistic understanding of health in the context of Grenada. We realized that we did not need to do housekeeping but to change and reorganize the system. We saw health not as a tokenism but as an investment in the development of Grenada.[70]

Thus after a thorough assessment of the inadequacies of the inherited system, the PRG engaged in the rebuilding of the health sector. This included repairs to existing facilities, establishment of more PHC centres and training of health personnel particularly those in primary and preventive care. In the 1981 New Year Address to the nation, one year after the revolution, Maurice Bishop (then the Minister of Health as well as the Prime Minister) outlined some of the gains achieved in health care.

> The revolution's most impressive advances in 1980 were in the areas of public health and popular education. Thousands of poor and working people benefited directly from these gains. For the first time in our history, the masses can now enjoy free basic medical care at governmental hospitals, clinics and health stations around the country. Instead of one clinic as before the revolution, our people now have the services of seven dental clinics, one for each parish. Over forty persons are now being treated daily by eye specialists at the Eye Clinic, and for the people of Petit Martinique, (PM) 1980 produced regular and very often weekly visits of doctors and dentists. We can state with pride and satisfaction that in 1980, over 50 thousand Grenadians received various forms of free medical care from our patriotic Grenadian doctors, some of whom returned to the homeland since the revolution, and from the hard working Cuban doctors, who in the true spirit of internationalism are assisting our revolution.[71]

The PRG administration, however, did not deal with the concerns of nurses immediately; these were not recognized until the nurses joined collectively and brought their case to Bishop. According to a senior nursing official,

> [d]uring a process of "peaceful negotiation" the nurses were able to open up areas of communication with the administration which before were impossible. This allowed for a more open and trusting climate to develop.[72]

Figure 7.1
Map of Grenada:
Location of Health Centres and Other Health Facilities

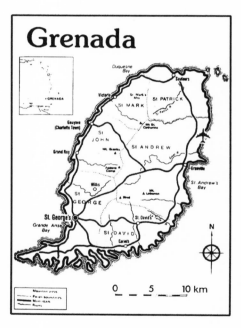

Health Districts	St. George	St. John	St. Mark	St. Patrick	St. Andrew	St. David	Carriacou & P.M.
Health Centres	1	1	-	1	1	1	1
Health Stations	9	2	1	4	4	3	4

A decentralized, well integrated system developed under the PRG. Primary care centres were enhanced to provide new and better services in the capital as well as in the rural areas, and all PHC services were coordinated in some way to SHC and THC services. Secondary and tertiary care were offered at the General Hospital in St. George; Princess Alice Hospital and Princess Royal Hospital (the two subsidiary hospitals), and a newly established hospital in Carriacou. Tertiary care was also provided by other institutions. (See Figure 7.1, Map of Grenada and Table 7.2)

As with Barbados, further examination of the Grenadian health care system will focus on the primary health care sector. The PHC services were provided by general practitioners through 5 health centres, 23 health stations and out-patient departments in the 3 general hospitals. The health centres which are equivalent to the Barbadian polyclinics, are normally run by trained nurse/midwives and provide a range of services. The health stations, also staffed by trained nurses, offer only basic services and are located in rural areas within a three mile radius of a village. Doctors only visit these stations once a week, at which time clinics are provided. The services offered at the health centres and health stations include: the daily dressings, ante-natal clinic, child welfare clinic, District Medical Officer"s clinic, immunization, domiciliary midwifery, and home visiting. Those offered only at health centres are the post-natal clinic, clinic for sexually transmitted diseases, psychiatric clinic, dental clinic, diabetes clinic, and hypertension clinic.[73]

Health Care Financing

Under the Gairy administration, about 70-75 percent of the 1978 health budget was invested in the three hospitals, while the remaining 25-30 percent of the budget was spent to service the 35 health centres and medical clinics around the country. Prime Minister Bishop stated that

> the obvious disadvantage to this approach is that the three areas of greater spending are precisely the areas that were attending to a very small percentage of those in our country who needed medical attention.[74]

Reports claimed that in order to correct this situation, the PRG began to invest more of the health budget in PHC, specifically in health education and promotion, rebuilding, and personnel retraining and training. By 1980 and 1981, health was receiving the second largest share of the current budget with 15 2/3 percent or EC $10.5 million (the largest share, 22 percent, was allocated to education).[75] In 1981 and 1982, the health budget as a percentage of the GDP was 4.9 percent and 5.0 percent respectively; this was equivalent to approximately 14.7 percent of the total government budget. (See Table 7.3)

Table 7.2
Health Facilities in Grenada and its Sister Islands

Facilities	Grenada	Carriacou	Petit Martinique	Total
Health Centres	5	1	—	6
Health Stations	23	3	1	27
Hospitals	3	1	—	4
Other Institutions*	5	—	—	5
Dispensaries	10	2	—	12
Laboratories	3	—	—	3

*These are all located in St. George and include: the Tuberculosis Sanitorium (25 beds); the Geriatric Home (137 beds); the Kennedy Home (for the handicapped; 16 beds); the Carlton Centre (for Alcoholism & Drug abuse; 16 beds).

Source: Harney, Lenore, "Grenada Health Situation Analysis," PAHO/WHO, September-October 1985, p. 67.

The rejuvenation process in the health care industry was facilitated by consultant expertise and financial and material assistance obtained from various regional and international sources. These included the Cuban Medical Brigade of over twenty doctors which began its work in June 1979; the World Pan-American Health Organization (PAHO); the World Health Organization (WHO); the Caribbean Common Market (CARICOM); the US Agency for International Development (USAID) which provided funding for refurbishing of the health centres; the Government of Venezuela; and the European Development Fund which provided funding for the construction of new health centres.[76] There was also the expansion of the operating facilities at the St. George"s General Hospital, the distribution of free milk in schools and communities and the nationwide organization of health education programmes. In summing up the development in health care delivery, De Riggs made note that the "massive level of free, voluntary, community participation in the refurbishing of the [health] centres"[77] had saved the government thousands of dollars. There was also an increase in the number of registered nurses, public health officers, community health aides, health education officers, nutrition assistants, pharmacists and laboratory technicians.

The fundamental result of all this development was country-wide free medical coverage for the first time in the history of Grenada. In addition, the quality of health facilities had improved greatly, as had the level of "health-community interdependence and inter-relation; and this made health care more available and accessible to the poor."[78] Alleyne also supported these claims, and noted that

> [c]ommunity health in Grenada was in general more than lip service to the Declaration of the Alma-Ata Conference, much more than revolutionary rhetoric....Health had been set as a national priority and this is evidenced by the allocation in the national budget to this sector.[79]

Perhaps the most significant observation was made by De Riggs, who acknowledged that the psychological well-being of the population was equally as important as their physical well-being.

> The absence of the terror of Gairyism has brought about a positive psychological change in our people. Much of the apathy, frustration and bewilderment has disappeared; a new spirit of buoyancy has pervaded the atmosphere in our country."[80]

Improved health care under the PRG could not have been achieved without the financial and human resources provided by the Cuban government, regional and international bodies and funding agencies. However, health care was not limited to the improvement of the infrastructure and services but in restoring the psycho-social well-being of the nation which was lacking during the GULP years.

Table 7.3
Grenada, Selected Health Economic Indicators
($ EC Millions)

	1974	1975	1976	1977	1978	1979	1980	1981	1982	1983
Total Governement Budget	20.2	24.1	36.0	32.2	45.2	53.4	59.6	66.9	66.9	79.8
Health & Housing Budget	3.2	3.6	4.8	5.4	6.9	7.6	8.6	10.2	9.8	11.2
% of Total Government Budget spent on Health & Housing	15.8	14.9	13.3	16.8	15.3	14.2	14.4	15.2	14.6	14.0
% of Total Government Budget spent on Health	—	—	—	—	—	—	—	14.7	14.7	13.6
Health expenditure as a % of GDP	—	—	—	—	—	—	—	4.9	5.0	5.1
Health expenditure per capita	—	—	—	—	—	—	—	93	98	100

Sources: (1) Harney, Lenore, "Grenada Health Situation Analysis", PAHO/WHO, September-October 1985, p.58; (2) Pyror, Frederic, Revolutionary Grenada: A Study in Political Economy, 1986, p.328.

Health Policy and Administration

Prime Minister Bishop, while attending his first meeting of CARICOM Health Ministers, stated:

> The People's Revolutionary Government of Grenada views health as a basic human right and as a funda-

mental prerequisite for the formulation of a sound economic policy.

The PRG health policy could be defined as multi-faceted; one which concurrently attacked both social and economic issues. For example, the government not only initiated free medical and dental care within the social services, but also addressed issues of formal and non-formal education, the building and repairing of low-cost housing and community centres and the improvement of transportation facilities to the rural communities.[81]

De Riggs claimed that one aim of the revolution was to demystify and democratize the system of medicine and health care. Thus, in the development of its first Three Year Heath Plan (1982 to 1985) for Grenada, Carriacou and Petit Martinique, the PRG government made sure that an inclusive approach to policy development was set in place, encouraging the active participation of the public and thereby ensuring that a "bottom-up" process was implemented. This strategy was confirmed by a senior public servant who stated:

> In doing the plan we went chapter by chapter, everybody read it, the nurses, the community. Although we did not reap the benefits [because of the Revolution"s demise].... [i]t is a document of good, hard, intensive work, the community participated in the true concept of community development.[82]

The Revolution's approach to health was based on the PHC concept. The objective was to have fewer people ill enough to require sophisticated and expensive hospital treatment, and in order to promote this new way of thinking, greater emphasis was placed on health education at the grass roots level, in health centres, workplaces and schools. Major additions to the health care system were the health service and health education programs provided specifically to organized workers; under this new scheme, sanitation and agricultural workers were entitled to medical and physical fitness examinations twice a year.

Establishment of the PHC model

Although the revolution sought to improve the overall services at the hospital, both in terms of personnel and equipment, its major focus was on the development of a primary health care system. The PHC was based on the "Alma Ata" concept which promoted an integrative approach to planning and involved the increased participation of other non-health care sectors.

> The primary health care model was revolutionary in concept. It redefined health and health policy; instead of viewing them as discrete entities, it incorporated everything impacting on individual and community well-being. It also emphasised local solutions using local resources, and therefore de-emphasised the role of medical professionals in local health care. It acknowledged the importance of traditional practitioners. The stress on local control and decision-making challenged the predominant top-down mechanisms of control, and pointed towards the development of a more egalitarian society. [83]

As noted by Stock and Aniyinam, the PHC model adopted by Grenada was not new but had been adapted from "the barefoot doctor model" which was successful in China and was subsequently introduced into other socialist countries (Cuba, Tanzania, and Mozambique). The adoption of the "authentic" model of the PHC seemed to be the natural path of development for the "socialist PRG" since their philosophy was to democratize the health services through the involvement of people. The PRG had not "developed legalistic attitudes to providing care to community people," [84] and this set them apart from some of their neighbours who had also adopted the PHC model. In order to ensure community participation and change people"s behaviors, the PRG government, according to a former Permanent Secretary, focused on

> the reconditioning of people into the preventative aspects of health rather than the curative and trying to get people to understand how you shift resources in order to introduce PHC in the health care system.[85]

Development of Health Care Teams

As mentioned, under the PRG, the health care system became more decentralized and community focused. This was evidenced by the formation of the primary PHC teams in each parish (one of the outstanding organizational features of the Grenada system). Each team had representatives from all sectors of health care, including environmental workers and maintenance workers. The team leaders from each team formed a unit whose task was to ensure coordination and reduce duplication in service delivery. Community health aides (CHA), a new category of health workers, were also represented on the teams. Eight CHAs, one from each parish, were selected and given a specifically designed program of preparation and their job was basically to

> work as part of the health team educating and inform-
> ing people about aspects of their health and also as the
> "front-line" of introduction to the health care system. [86]

The CHAs were successful as a link between the professional health care team and the community; "because they were well-known and easily accepted, the message got in and out in a much more effective way.[87]

The development of PHC was described as unique within the Grenadian context because it allowed the interaction of people from across all sectors and promoted the removal of social and racial barriers in the society. This change was succinctly described by a former government official.

> When we got the PHC teams implemented, people
> began looking at other health care workers as people,
> as persons; they cooperated because they understood
> what we were trying to achieve. Lack of information was
> one of the biggest killers in our society, when people
> don't know why things are done, and they don't know
> how and nobody communicates with them and make
> them feel that they are making a contribution. During
> the PRG days the street cleaners were waving when
> you passed because they felt happy to be recognized as
> a member of the health team. Previous to that when
> health workers passed they turned their car windows
> up because they were doing filthy work and dirty work.[88]

Throughout the rebuilding process, the PHC teams monitored the entire public health system on a quarterly basis. The monitoring activity was described by the above government official as one which

> involved all the "chief" (senior) technocrats and professionals at the Ministry of Health. We then went into the districts to meet with the teams and to see how they were doing, to look at their performance, to look at their targets, if they achieved, how they achieved and if they didn"t, why not. All the chiefs were there to deal with specific problems related to their specific areas and that kind of link was necessary in order to allow cohesiveness to the whole approach. We were not sitting here reading reports when in reality the situation out there was something else.[89]

A second monitoring system, which worked in collaboration with the Ministry of Health, was also in place at the district or village level.

> The district group or village groups were political groups but they looked at problems related to that particular community or that particular parish. From time to time we would be called in if there was a particular health problem to discuss it and to listen to it. So there was another monitoring system outside of the health system to give us feedback.[90]

This informal route proved to be indispensable to the Ministry because they were provided with "information that normally would not come through the system."[91] This was beneficial for planning as well as evaluating the progress of the programmes.

Human Resources Planning

During the 1979 to 1983 period, the government focused on the training and retraining of health care providers at all levels and, by 1981, they had a comprehensive array of professionals. (See Table 7.4 a & 7.4 b for human resources figures)

The Cuban government not only helped to finance the education and training of Grenadians, but also supplied a team of medical doctors and specialists (the "Cuban Brigade") who were assigned to the hospitals as well as to the clinics and assisted with the implementation of the PHC programme. Although there was an immediate need for health personnel (created by the emigration of "trained professionals" to the better working conditions of the developed countries), the training and retraining of health personnel was not performed on an ad hoc basis. Rather, the government attempted to address the country's long term health manpower needs in a more organized way through the assistance given by the Cuban government and by encouraging Grenadians living abroad and other non-Grenadians to work in Grenada. The strategy was explained in this way:

> During the period we were able to focus on the issues in a more intensive way as part of our human resource development plan,.... we sat down and said.... we want to achieve a certain ratio between doctors and people.... so that we could look down the road and say, if we send so many people to train in Cuba as doctors then in seven years the government would be less dependent on the whims and fancies of some of the doctors.... there was a traditional kind of aura, prestige and mysticism about doctors and medicine and.... the revolution was going to break that, we realized that we were treading on the corns of the old establishment of the medical professionals, but this was part of the revolution,.... we were interested in solving our medical staff requirements, our specialist staff requirements, and we saw it as part of our manpower planning and development, as human resource development, and we sent people to train, large number of doctors to train as specialists.[92]

According to Maurice Bishop, this increased the available physician manpower.

> There are now forty doctors and seven dentists providing free medical care to 110,000 people in Free and Revolutionary Grenada. In 1979 the figures stood at twenty-three doctors and one dentist. The present ratio is 1 doctor to under 3000 people and 1 dentist to 16,000 people. Before March 13th, 1979 the ratio was 1 doctor to 4000 people and 1 dentist to 28,000.[93]

Other health personnel also benefited from the training programs and their numbers increased. In addition, as indicated earlier, new positions were developed in an effort to better service the general public. Health education programmes established were facilitated by health educators and community outreach was achieved through the community health aides and the district nurses who traveled into rural areas to deliver care.

A number of personnel were, however, in disagreement with these new training practices of the PRG and with the immigration policies, specifically as they related to "the influx of foreign trained doctors" into Grenada. In regard to the situation as it related to physicians, one particular doctor felt that

> [d]uring the revolution people were trained as doctors who did not have the basic qualifications needed to go to university. We had only a mediocre system.... It was necessary for the revolution to show that they were doing something so there were numbers but the services were inappropriate... Unfortunately most of the doctors who came were inappropriate. As far as I am concerned health care in Carriacou never improved any great deal from Gairy time to the PRG time. In the PRG time there were just numbers but they were inappropriate.[94]

Another member of the medical profession claimed that

> In Grenada they had adjusted their registration system to allow the Cuban doctors to be able to practice... Also there were signs of discontent coming from the local medical personnel who felt that Cuban doctors were given special privileges and were being paid very well. It was felt that if this same money was used to upgrade the local doctors' salaries in the government services they would have had a better service.[95]

This feeling of displeasure from among some members of the medical profession against both the Cuban doctors and Cuban-trained doctors was both an ideological reaction as well as a snobbish attitude that is prevalent among Western-trained doctors. The allegation of paying salaries to Cuban doctors was denied by the former Deputy Minister of Health who claimed "that it was the Cuban Government who supported the Grenada Health Care system and not the other way around.[96]

On the other hand, there were some personnel who were quite complimentary of the PRG's efforts. A senior official who "was a product" of specialist training, noted that the

> 1979 to 83 period could be seen as the "evolution" of training in Grenada. A number of people who did not have the personal financial resources to afford tertiary level training, particularly outside of the country were given an opportunity.... If you look at the present health care system, you will find that the backbone of the system are people who were trained under the PRG.[97]

In addition, the PRG"s training policies were highly regarded since they not only created educational opportunities through scholarships, but also allowed for a planned process of human resources development not only in the health sectors but in other areas as well.

SUMMARY

During the 1979 to 1983 period, Grenada was governed by a socialist regime that attempted to modify the country"s economy by pursuing "a mixed" economic model. Under the PRG it nevertheless remained largely dependent on external financing and was susceptible to unstable market prices.

Through the mass mobilization and participation of various groups, the PRG was successful in implementing a number of social programs to improve the well-being of the population. The NWO, for example, was instrumental in organizing women "in the process of the revolution" and ensuring that gender inequality became an issue. Despite these gains, however, women were largely under-represented at the ultimate decision-making levels.

The PHC is another example of the power of interdisciplinary teams and community involvement. Introduced through the establishment of primary health teams, the PHC promoted a change in the population"s thinking from a medical to a preventative perspective, and shifts in resource allocation supported this challenge. Whether the system truly supported women"s health issues or whether women were merely used as tools (productive roles) to achieve the PRG"s revolutionary goals is debatable and will be further investigated through the interviews with administrators, providers and working class women themselves.

Table 7.4 a
Manpower (Grenada):
Health Personnel with Population Ratio, 1981

Category	Total	Ratio/10,000
Hospital Administrator & Project Officer	2	18.0
Doctors, including District Medical Officer (D.M.O)	38	3.5
Nurses, including Public Health Nurses (P.H.A),	138	13.0
District Nurse/midwives (N/M)		
and Family Nurse Practitioners (F.N.P.)		
Nursing Assistants	21	1.9
Nursing Attendants	127	11.9
Community Health Aides (C.H.A)	44	4.1
Student Nurse	82	7.7
Dietitian/Nutritionist	*	*
Health Educator	1	.09
Social Worker	*	*
Physiotherapist	2	0.1
Environmental Health Officer (E.H.O)	31	2.9
Dentist & Dental Auxiliaries	3	0.2
Pharmacist, Radiographer,	19	1.7
Lab technologist/technician		
Medical Record Officer & Statistician	1	.09

Table 7.4 b
Manpower Distribution (Grenada): Health Personnel Per Health District, 1981

Health District	P.H.N.	Dist. N/M	C.H.A.	D.M.O.	Phar.	F.N.P.	E.H.O.
St. George	2	8	13	4	4	*	5
St. John/ St. Mark	1	3	4	1	1	1	5
St. Patrick	1	5	5	1	1	1	1
St. Andrew	1	5	6	1	1	1	1
St. David	1	4	8	1	1	1	1
Carriacou & Petit Martinique	1	2	5	1	1	1	1

* Not Available

Source: Harney, Lenore. "Grenada Health Situation Analysis.": PAHO/WHO, September-October 1985, pp. 64 & 86.

Notes

1. See Didacus Jules. "Education and Social Transformation in Grenada 1979-1983." Madison: Ph.D dissertation, University of Winconsin, 1992; see also Ambursley (1984); Brizan (1979).
2. See George Brizan. Grenada - Island of Conflict: From Amerindian to Peoples Revolution 1498-1979 London (ed.) Press, 1984.
3. Ibid.:329.
4. Ibid.:332.
5. Ibid; see also Fitzroy Ambursley & James Dunkerley (1984).
6. George Brizan (1984):333.
7. Ibid.
8. Ibid.:337.
9. See Fitzroy Ambursley & Robin Cohen (eds) Crisis in the Caribbean New York: Monthly Review Press, 1983.
10. Anne Walker. "Grenada's Women-Four Years after March 1979." Caribbean Contact: 1983:12; see also Ambursley & Dunkerley (1984).
11. Fitzroy Ambursley & James Dunkerley (1984):26.
12. Carl Stone, Power in the Caribbean Basin: A Comparative Study of Political Economy: InterAmerican Political Series, 1984 :40, see also Fitzroy Ambursley (1984).
13. See Fitzroy Ambursley & James Dunkerley (1984)
14. Ibid.
15. Fitzroy Ambursley & James Dunkerley. Grenada Whose Freedom.

New York: Latin American Bureau, 1984:27.

16. Didacus Jules. (1992) pp:147-148.
17. Fitzroy Ambursley & James Dunkerley (1984):28.
18. Ibid.
19. See Fitzroy Ambursley & Robin Cohen. (1983); Jules (1992).
20. Fitzroy Ambursley & James Dunkerley. (1984):29.
21. Didacus Jules. (1992):139.
22. See Fitzroy Ambursley & James Dunkerley. (1984).
23. Carl Stone "Democracy and the State: The Case of Jamaica." The State in Caribbean Society . Mona, Jamica: Department of Economics, UWI, 1986:38; see also Fitzroy Ambursley & James Dunkerley (1984).
24. Fitzroy Ambursley & James Dunkerley. (1984) pp:32-33.
25. Didacus Jules (1992):149; see also Brian Meeks (1991); and Manning Marable (1987).
26. Fitzroy Ambursley & James Dunkerley (1984):30.
27. See Didacus Jules (1992); Fitzroy Ambursley & James Dunkerley (1984); and others.
28. See Ambursley & Dunkerley (1984); Didacus Jules (1992); Don Rojas (1982).
29. Fitzroy Ambursley & James Dunkerley. (1984): 37.
30. See Fitzroy Ambursley & Robin Cohen. (1983).
31. Fitzoy Ambursley & James Dunkerley. (1984):208.
32. See Fitzroy Ambursley & James Dunkerley. (1984).
33. Ibid.:40.
34. Didacus Jules. (1992):177.
35. See Lewis E David. (1984).
36. See Didacus Jules. (1992).
37. Current economic position and prospects for Grenada, 1979, Latin America and Caribbean Regional Office, World Bank quoted by Ambursley, "Grenada the New Jewel Movement" in Ambursley Fitzroy and Cohen Robin, (eds) Crisis in the Caribbean, New Yorks Monthly Review Press, 1983:199.
38. Ambursley, Fitzroy "Wither Grenada? An Investigation into the March 13th Revolution One Year After" Society's in Crisis;1980:433.
39. See Fitzroy Ambursley & Robin Cohen. (1983); Fitzroy Ambursley (1980).
40. Fitzroy Ambursley. (1983).
41. Didacus Jules (1992) pp:159-160.
42. Coard quoted by Fitzroy Ambursley. (1983) pp:203-204.
43. Fitzroy Ambursley & James Dunkerley. (1984):204.
44. Coard quoted by Ambursley. (1983):204.
45. Didacus Jules (1992):178; see also Fitzroy Ambursley & James Dunkerley (1984).

46. Ambursley, Fitzroy, and Cohen, Robin (1983):206.
47 Ibid.
48. Ibid.
49. Ibid.
50. Ibid.:208.
51. Ann Walker. (1983):12.
52. Didacus Jules. (1992):184.
53. Didacus Jules. (1992).
54. See Jocelyn Massiah, 1986.
55. Bishop quoted by Didacus Jules. (1992):184.
56. Interview, October 1992.
57. James Ferguson (1980); see also Didacus Jules. (1992).
58. Bishop quoted by Didacus Jules. (1992) pp:184-185.
59. Rita Joseph. (1981):17.
60. Rosemary Ann Porter "Women and the State: women's movements in Grenada and their role in Grenadian revolution 1979-1983" (PhD dissertation, Temple University, 1986):407.
61. Ibid.
62. Ibid.
63. Coard, Phyllis, quoted by Didacus Jules (1992):157; see also Dessima Williams (1992).
64. See Rita Joseph (1981); see also Jules (1992); James Ferguson (1990); Kathy Sunshine (1982); Anne Walker (1983) and EPICA (1984).
65. Rosemary Ann Porter (1986).
66. Didacus Jules (1992):186.
67. Rosemary Ann Porter (1986):79.
68. Chris De Riggs, Deputy Minister of Health "Health Care: Achievements and Prospects" 1981:73.
69. Interview, October 1992.
70. Ibid.
71. "Address by Prime Minister Bishop on Primary Health Care in the parish of St David's" The Free West Indian, October 24, 1981 pp:1-2.
72. Interview, October 1992.
73. See Lenore Harney: PAHO/WHO, September-October 1985:71.
74. The Free West Indian;1981 pp:4-5.
75. See Didacus Jules (1992).
76. See Davis, 1984; see also Chris De Riggs (1981).
77. Chris De Riggs (1981):75.
78. Davis (1984).
79. Candia Alleyne, "Changing Perspectives in Health Care Development in Grenada." Bulletin of Eastern Caribbean Affairs: March - April 1981: 17.
80. Chris De Riggs (1981):75.

81. James Ferguson (1990) pp:80-81;*see* also Didacus Jules (1992).
82. Interview, October 1992.
83. V.Sidel and R. Sidel quoted by Stock and Anyinam (1992).
84. Interiew, October 1992.
85. Ibid.
86. Ibid.
87. Ibid.
88. Ibid.
89. Ibid.
90. Ibid.
91. Ibid.
92. Ibid.
93. Chris De Riggs. "Achievements and Prospects." Grenada is not alone-speeches by the PRG at the 1st International Conference in Solidarity with Grenada. St. George's: Fedon Publishers, November 1981 pp:74-75; *see* also Clive Thomas (1988) and Michael Aberdeen (1984).
94. Interview, October 1992.
95. Interview, November 1992.
96. Ibid.
97. Interview, October 1992.

CHAPTER 8

Assessment of State Health Care in Barbados and Grenada: The Professional's Perspective

The previous two chapters examined the political, socio-economic and health policies of Barbados and Grenada individually. Tentative conclusions were formulated about how these systems affected the operations of the PHC and the delivery of gender-sensitive services. This chapter gives a comparison of the state policies of Barbados and Grenada in relation to health care as articulated by the bureaucracy and others in authority.

One objective of this study was to determine whether the documented health policies of the two countries were actually implemented through health care programs that effectively addressed the primary health care needs of women, particularly working-class women. So far, an analysis of historical and other secondary data sources would indicate that the issue of women's health was not a priority of either the BLP or the PRG. To determine whether this was the case or not, providers and health care administrators and policy makers in each country were asked to critique their respective health care systems during the 1979 to 1983 period and to note if there were any subsequent changes. Their responses, which were grouped under several categories,[1] are presented below.

GENDER SENSITIVITY

The professionals differed in their views with respect to the degree of sensitivity shown by the state towards women's health issues. There were some who felt that the state was aware of and responsive to the health needs of women, as did this senior Barbadian civil servant:

> I think government [DLP] is highly sensitive to the needs of women and in particular to their health status in terms of their maternal/reproductive roles. A lot of work has been done, but they need, through the analysis, to be made aware of the new areas of concerns of women. For example, the areas of chemicals, that everybody is at risk.... Both governments [BLP and DLP] have placed a major focus on women's health but new things come along.[2]

A senior Barbadian nursing officer also agreed that both governments had addressed women's health:

> I would say that both governments have concentrated on women's health. I would say that the services have expanded a lot in areas such as pap smears, breast examinations and family planning services.

A Grenadian public servant also gave his perspective of the PRG's policies on women's health:

> I would say that the PRG was sensitive to women's health. I would say yes from three points of view. One from the fact that in the health care system, you find that women were in the majority, in terms of givers of health care and the fact that government, at that time, took time out to analyze the needs of the people who were actually delivering the health and try to meet some of those needs. I think that gives clear evi-

dence of its commitment to the development of women in that level. Secondly, we had at that time a vibrant national women's organization, which I think articulated the needs of women quite categorically and mass mobilization of women and they addressed the needs of women at all levels, professional women, working class women etc. Thirdly, in the aspect of maternal and child health, I think, we all know that the whole business of child bearing, which although sad is true, is left solely in many occasions to the responsibility of the woman. The PRG made a special effort to develop maternal and child health facilities to meet the needs of women who were not able to come into St. George's to have a baby, so we had the birth of rural maternal and child health complexes in all the parishes. So because these facilities were made available to rural women, again that says how conscious the government was at that particular period in relationship to the needs of women in reproductive and other roles. From an educational standpoint the PRG broke the barriers from what we called the traditional roles of women in our society....I think that was the era when the women of Grenada started to become aware of who they were, of what your role in society was.[3]

And although women's health was not a major organizing strategy of the NWO, this is what a former NWO representative had to say,

I won't say that we didn't organize around health. We didn't organize women around health issues but we did take up health issues. For example the Depo Provera contraceptive injection. A lot of women were complaining about the effects of it. We met with the Ministry of Health and the Family Planning Association and stopped the Family Planning Association from bringing it in. We made a big issue of it. This drug was banned in North America and why are they bringing it to the Third World. During the PRG time it became illegal to use the drug. We did a lot of education around it; we were not against family planning but we were against that particular contraception. We held discussions and we organized at the national level and got different health professional to go into the district to talk about it.[4]

What is clearly apparent from these comments made by both Barbadian and Grenadian officials is that women are still viewed reproductively (and productively, in the case of Grenada), rather than holistically and hence there is a definite focus on those aspects of their health. It is, however, fair to say that the Barbadian official recognized this weakness in the system, and to acknowledge the PRG for making some strides in terms of health education and promotion.

On the other end of the spectrum, there were professionals from both countries who felt that their respective systems were insensitive to the health concerns and issues of women. For example, a senior Barbadian politician stated that personally, in terms of his portfolio, he was sensitive to the needs of women, but in terms of his government he stated:

I would have to say I don't think so. I don't think the administration as such of health-the people across the board who are the managers of the Health Care system perceive women's health as a subject.... although I would say that Barbados is further ahead as compared with other Caribbean territories in this concept of women's health.[5]

Similarly a senior Grenadian civil servant claimed, in reference to the 1979 to1983 period, that "there was no specific policy made with any particular reference to women."[6] This was supported by a Grenadian family physician who claimed that neither the PRG (1979 to 1983), nor the present National Democratic Congress (NDC)

has been sensitive to women's health issues. Not to any significant degree, I don't think so, on health as a general perspective but not on women's health. I have not been aware of this by any administration.[7]

With respect to the NDC's stance on the issue, a senior

Grenadian government official acknowledged that the government,

> recognize[d] health as an important issue but that's all there is to it, a recognition.... It [Women's Affairs] is no longer a department. We have absolutely no budget. We have tried to get some external funding through writing proposals and we hope we can get funding. We have not gone into the area of health. There is supposed to be a Health Desk in the Ministry of Health in which women's affairs should have played a focal role; that is not happening. We had attempted to have an inter-ministerial group so that we could bring in those sectors like Health, Agriculture and other areas but we were not able to do that either, so health generally is getting a low priority.[8]

Another Grenadian, a former senior government employee, articulated the same sense of loss, confusion and lack of coordination in the health care system since the demise of the PRG.

> You have a lot of situations now that women don't know where to go, where to turn to for help. I know for sure that hypertension is one of the major problems because women are under a lot of stress. I am saddened because there is no focus on health right now.... You get slogans coming from the Ministry of Health saying Health For All by the Year 2000, these broad statements but I am not aware there is any main thrust into focusing on the health of women or providing services. From the way we are going we may all be dead by the Year 2000.[9]

Still, a large number of the providers were of the opinion that the health care system should be neutral and unbiased, objectively based on diagnosis and treatment of disease pattern and not on gender. These gender-blind views were expressed not only by the men but were also voiced by several female health providers at all levels of the hierarchy. At the clinical level, as articulated by this senior Barbadian public health nurse, specific attention was not paid to women as a whole.

We would be inclined to say not women's health, we need health care for men and women, both sides.... we can't look at women, we have to look at families.[10]

This gender-neutral view of health care was also evident at the higher administrative level, as expressed by this senior Barbadian hospital administrator who felt that

[t]he question of women's health is a perceptual need. I think it is difficult to single out women's health in that way. For example cancer is the number one killer. This is recognized and pap smears are provided. Those programs are very successful. The use of information was not because we, singled them out because they are women but because it is a 'high risk." There are interest groups who protect their own needs as they see it.... I don't think that male problems are dealt with to the exclusion of women's problems. I think a lot of it depends on the prominence attached to the particular disease entity and if you have a gynaecologist who is interested in women or men, then that gets pushed.... I find some difficulty myself in determining if treatment of disease is sexist.[11]

These systemic views were also evident at the ministerial level, as this following quote by a senior Barbadian Ministry of Health official indicates:

I can't agree that women's health care has not been a priority. There is accessibility of care regardless of class, creed, gender and social status. We cannot say that attention has not been paid to women. Lots of money has been spent. The problem is designing health care for any gender is disease analysis. If the problem confronting us is disease X, then we provide care for disease X. Health is provided in the context we can plan in the Ministry of Health. Women in the Caribbean have always had care.[12]

These claims for neutrality in the delivery of health services are in fact flawed. Research shows that not only can the same treatments have different outcomes on the two sexes because of their physiology, but that men and women may be treated differently for the same disease, not because of the manifestation of the disease and their physiological make-up, but because of the difference in gender. For example, research has found that a consistently higher proportion of women than men received tranquilizers and that women continued to use the drug for longer periods than their male counterparts.[13] Other research shows that young women are under represented in pre-marketing drug trials and that the reasons for exclusion "include the additional problem of analyzing data, women's tendency to report adverse reactions more frequently than men, and the shifts in women's hormonal cycle."[14] Achilles argues that "if the research samples for the testing of a particular drug are limited to one sex or the other or fails to monitor the difference in responses between sexes, the (safe) recommended dosages or studies of side effects will be unreliable."[15] Generally, according to Clement, research shows "that physicians as a group, treat male and female clients differently,"[16] thus whether the women's health issues are regarded as separate, specific areas of focus or concern, the treatment women receive differs from that delivered to men, simply because they are women.

BARRIERS TO HEALTH CARE SERVICES

The view that women's health does not deserve priority or that health services should not be gendered has created several barriers which have limited the accessibility and availability of services to working class women and thus the overall quality of their health. The obstacles include middle class women in positions of power, ability to pay for services, the attitudes of service providers, the relationship between doctors and nurses, the relationship between hospital and polyclinic nurses and the lack of consumer involvement in activities involving their own health. Each "barrier" to appropriate, timely service will be discussed individually.

Middle Class Women

The senior staff of the Barbados Ministry of Health in 1992 consisted of four women who held the positions of Permanent Secretary, Chief Medical Officer of Health and Senior Medical Officers of Health; women were also represented in the administrative and technical areas of the Ministry. The view was that since women were in strategic "power" positions, they could influence policies that affected women. This perception is flawed since it is not necessarily true that women in the bureaucracy are automatically supportive of issues which may associate them with "feminist" concerns or may be familiar with issues facing working class women, being mostly middle class themselves. This fact was substantiated by two sources:

A senior international health official explained that

> [w]omen in the Ministries were often the biggest stumbling blocks, they see no need for a special emphasis on women's health. Some of them say "look at me I have made it through the system, women don't need any special attention." It was far easier to get one of the males to sit down and discuss the Health, Women and Development Plan than it is to get women in the Health Ministries to listen to you. In one Ministry the women laughed at me-what nonsense are you talking about; three senior women professionals.[17]

A regional NGO representative supported the above claim, stating that

> A lot of women who are in certain positions have never looked beyond their domestic help; their life is not stressful because other women have taken care of their domestic chores. Because of their education they can divorce themselves from what is happening.[18]

This lack of awareness/sensitivity by women in management position and by the bureaucracy was confirmed by more than one senior health official; the official line was "our mandate is family health, not women's health. We can't look at women, we have to look at families." This statement is not only a denial of reality but is unrealistic especially in the context of the Caribbean where the majority of families are single-parented and female-headed.[19]

Ability to Pay for Services

According to a senior Barbadian health official, the provision of health care is related to one's economic situation. The attitude of Barbadian providers towards system users varies according to the user's ability to pay for services regardless of whether those people are considered poor people. In elaborating on this point, he made use of a hypothetical comparison between services offered by a private practitioner and those services offered at the government facilities.

> At the private clinic the person is known as Mr. X. The person who attends the public clinic is known as No. 2 . That person becomes dehumanized and is put off by that reception, regardless of how good the care is.[20]

The exact opposite was true of Grenada. Whereas Barbadians placed more value on fee-for-service care (because of the "poor" stigma associated with free services), the Grenadians were finding it difficult to accept fee-for-service care after the PRG days of free medical care.

A senior nutritionist declared that

> During the PRG money was not the focus but keeping people well, that was the focus. We were exposed to all dental treatment. Now you will have to pay if you want proper health care-you have to go to a private doctor.

A senior Grenadian health bureaucrat explained how the proposed 1992 cuts in health and fee-for-service would limit access to health care.

> The services under the PRG were free. We are also supposed to be giving free health care or the minimum but now because of the recession we cannot really give the standard and quantity we had hoped to; we were told to cut services, but the public has become accustomed to a certain quantity and so on....

We have had to send people abroad for treatment because we have had difficulty in recruiting people to man the service-staff.... We are trying to look at user fees but the policy may be difficult in the recession, people are out of work. To put a fee on now is hard, but we are trying to get back what we can from those we think can afford it, health insurance, etc.[21]

The Barbadians and Grenadians views on how "good" health care services should be delivered (free versus fee-for-service) differed significantly, a difference that could be attributed to the different ideological positions of the two States and their interpretation of the "right" to health care.

Attitude of Service Providers

A Barbadian ministry official claimed that they have tried to deal with the problem of provider attitudes towards non-paying clients by organizing several courses including a reorientation of the doctors and nurses to move away from the "Poor Law System" which provided care exclusively to the poor and indigent. The objective was to get the providers to think of their clients as "our people, our extended family instead of those people."[22] Personally, he felt that "the newer medical practitioners were not practicing holistic medicine.... and that older doctors generally took more time with the patients."[23]

Even though some attempts were made to address the issues of attitudinal change of the newer medical practitioners by the introduction of community health and a new program of community medical attachment for the new batch of internships, a senior administrator raised the concern that

[r]egrettably, one of the areas that is not satisfactory is that folks at the hospital see themselves as specialists and super specialists and the others out there as the ones who deal with basic care Public Health and so on. This comes about as a result of the teaching of the medical staff.[24]

This attitude of snobbishness among the medical hierarchy is evident among both doctors and nurses who are hospital-based and these findings were corroborated by two health care professionals, one of whom stated:

> First of all that attitude between primary care and secondary/tertiary care medicine exists long before someone becomes a doctor, it is ingrained from medical school. The people who are given the prestige within the university setting are the hospital consultants. There is rivalry even between medical doctors and surgeons.... that exists between the hospital and non-hospital people, but if 90% of your exposure is to the hospital then that is the "brain-washing" you will get. Also if the university training does not take public health, put it in a position in which it should be regarded and teach students the potential and importance that it has and the scope it should have, their minds are already made up; mind-sets already exist by the time you graduate. In fact there is a lot more community medicine being done now but even now that is still regarded by students as a nuisance that has to be got through so to speak, and the hospital consultants resent the community medicine and this is distinct from public health. The amount of public health remains unsatisfactory.... There is a sort of hierarchy where the hospital doctors feel they are best, then they may consider the general practitioner, then at the bottom is the polyclinic doctor.[25]

Although some steps have been taken to rectify the "attitude problem," according to a senior international health official, the "training of health personnel has not kept in line with the new acclaimed health policy"[26] and thus, professionals are not equipped to deliver community- based primary health care in the polyclinics. The professionals unanimously agreed that since the demise of the PRG, the attitude of providers had changed, negatively affecting their relationships with clients. A senior nurse worried about this.

> The relationship between the providers and users is not good now. People do their work and go home. They don't talk to patients. What is on your treatment card; if it is an injection, that is what they give,

there is no deeper relationship like before.[27]

A senior Grenadian health manager also found that provider attitudes had become a problem.

> Attitude now is a problem throughout the system as I see it sitting here. I do not know what has caused the change. What I mean is change is something that goes on all the time. We are working on helping the providers to appreciate the users; if they weren't there we would have no jobs. Many days I get a lot of complaints because there are always conflicts going on throughout the system. The attitude is not what we would like.[28]

A senior district nurse tried to explain the reasoning behind the attitudinal change:

> The attitudes of the providers have definitely changed. The incentives are not there so it brings about a relationship of not really caring. The attitude is if the patients don't care, why should the nurse.[29]

From the above comments, it is evident that efforts made to promote a patient-sensitive and focused care by the PRG have been reversed, creating a situation that negatively impacts on the delivery of health care.

Doctor-Nurse Relationships

One senior Barbadian public health nurse noted that the services had improved generally over the last ten years (1982 to 1992). However, she expressed dissatisfaction with regard to one development, the establishment of a delivery suite at the Queen Elizabeth Hospital.

> Ante-natal care has been taken from the nurses. Nurses used to do a lot of that care; that has been taken away, doctors are now doing it. I am a bit concerned because doctors never have the time to counsel and sit down and listen. They just look at the tummy. They would never ask about the toddler at

home or if they have any problems, and they were not geared for that, the nurses are trained for that. In that step it might be good for the woman on one part but she is missing something on the other part.[30]

It is evident from these statements that a power struggle exists between the nurses and doctors, with the latter (as is usually the case) infringing on the professional jurisdiction of the former. The nurse-doctor relationship was also said to be less than satisfactory during the PRG regime, with claims that the nurses were unhappy with the male chauvinism of the Cuban doctors.

The "poor" relationship between doctors and nurses is not unique to Barbados and Grenada but has to do with the way in which nurses (women) are viewed by the largely male-dominated medical profession. Despite the fact that nurses form the "backbone of the extensive primary health care in the Caribbean,"[31] it is the doctors (largely male) who have the prestige and power within these societies; and more and more, the professions which were normally the domain of women in the Caribbean are gradually being taken over by the predominantly male medical profession. For example, the role of the nurse-midwives who played a key role in the family care delivery system has not only become institutionalized and medicalized but the nursing profession is also being further relegated to "handmaidens" to the medical profession.[32]

State Hospital Nurse-Polyclinic Nurse Relationship

The emphasis on THC in Barbados is even evidenced in the relationships between hospital and Polyclinic nurses. As was pointed out, since the community health nurses are clinic-based, the clinic takes precedence over the community, causing valuable community resources and expertise to be under-utilized. One of the senior public health nurses described the relationship between state hospital and polyclinic nurses in Barbados as difficult since hospital- trained nurses saw themselves as more knowledgeable than nurses working in the public health sector. The situation she confessed, was

not as good as I would like to see it. For example you send a patient to hospital but you never know the outcome; very few doctors would send back the history note. Personally, if it is something special, you might call up and get some information. If the nurse on the other end doesn't really know you, you are not getting any information, never mind if you are a nurse or a supervisor; they tend to withhold information. A lot of times we have to depend on what the patient says and that to my mind is not good enough if it is something that needs to be looked at.... When we visited the hospital we were told that the mechanism was in place to deal with this problem but the mechanism has to be worked out by people; and if the people don't do it then it is not done.[33]

A Grenadian nurse described a similar strained relationship between the community and hospital personnel:

Presently, the relationship is not nice. We do not have conflict as such, but it should be better; the community and the hospital should relate more closely. We are not seeing that. Sometimes when you go there to borrow things they are not helpful. You find that once you no longer work within the hospital setting the nurses ostracize you. I don't know if they feel that we are not doing nursing anymore. Maybe they don't understand what community nursing really is. I think they need to educate the nurses at the hospital about what we do because we know what they are doing and not just the nurses but the administration as well.[34]

The inflexible working relationships that existed between the medical (hospital-based) sector and public health sector professionals (the situation was similar for doctors) obviously hampered the continuity and consistency of care delivered to the public at large.

Consumer Involvement

The PRG seemed to appreciate the value of empowering individuals and communities and allowing them to make informed decisions about their own health and to take an active role in shaping the delivery of health care. A Grenadian community worker reminisced:

> During the revolution, the masses were mobilized and
> they were prepared to work to build houses, schools,
> clinics because they knew they saw some benefits later
> on. In relation to health, everybody was involved. It
> was a political activity, everyone from the leadership
> down was involved. People participated because they
> saw the future benefits in terms of their own health
> and the health of their families. All that community
> spirit is now dead. You have to pay people now if you
> want to do community work. During the PRG people
> were also given things like milk, kerosene, etc.[35]

A former public servant also reflected on the PRG days and the
ability of women groups to mobilize efforts around community-
based programs:

> During the revolution, there was enough staff to con-
> centrate on programs in the villages-proper food,
> proper nutrition. Food supplements also were given
> at the time: butter, oil, milk and grain, corn and things
> like that. Then the women's groups really organized
> looking after those areas. After the invasion the whole
> program was sort of thrown out, we could not support
> it, the staff was cut.[36]

The Barbadians also realized the importance of consumer participation in health. However, the attempts made so far by the
government to encourage community participation in the development and management of services has been unsuccessful, an
outcome blamed on

> [a] certain mystique that still surrounds the delivery of
> health care in the community. For an improved health
> status of the country to be achieved, the total com-
> munity must shoulder its part of the load and partici-
> pate in the management of the health services.[37]

An NWO representative identified the behavior of those in power
as a major weakness of the health system, stating that greater
consumer involvement would require

both senior officials and ministers to change their behavior and to give up some of their power. The philosophy of primary health care is the empowering of people and one of the features of PHC is the development of "local health systems," and what that fundamentally means is the transfer of power from the centre to the periphery.[38]

In the arguments above it is obvious that not only the traditional definition of health is being applied, but also that the multi-dimensional roles performed by women[39] and the impact of these roles on their health are being ignored.[40] The majority of women are employed in jobs that are low paying and considered an extension of women's domestic roles. Reports have shown that women are more likely to be exposed to health hazards and risks from cleaning agents used both at home and in the workplace. In addition, the 'medical model' does not include other elements of women's lives and the stresses to which they may be exposed. For working class women, the literature submits "that the incidence of depression suggest that where the inequalities of class (and race) combine with those of gender, depression indeed appears to be an occupational hazard of caring."[41] For example, women often have to confront issues of poverty, sexism, sexual harassment, domestic violence and lack of support services. Of the professionals interviewed, three Barbadian women (one a physician and two NGO professionals) noted that a special emphasis should be placed on women's health. The family physician acknowledged that

> [a] lot of issues are overlooked, the roles women play as health providers, both in formal and informal settings are overlooked and in a certain sense under-utilized and in terms of their illnesses we definitely need to pay more attention to women and their problems.[42]

One of the NGO professionals' comments supported the above views:

> Women and men are not involved in the same kind of responsibilities. The realities of women's lives of having to work at home and go to work and then

return home to take care of the family is not the same for men. Men do not share in this experience and if they do it is only in the form of helping. The wear and tear on women bodies is not an experience men have, not just childbirth but all the demands that are made on women's lives, in terms of relatives and the community as well as the economic situation. Therefore their needs/demands are greater in health even though it may not show up in the statistics.[43]

The failure to view women's health holistically should not come as a surprise since Weinensee's observation is that "[w]hat has been traditionally accepted in western culture as health care in reality is medical "ill care."[44] She argues that "health professions are not conceptually well equipped to study health, that they have virtually no vocabulary or classification of functional capacity in health, and, while they have concentrated appropriately on the control and study of disease, they now must attend to positive health maintenance,"[45] and furthermore that even "nurses accept but do not strive for this positive goal. Instead they concern themselves with illness ... paying more attention to mal-adjustment and physical ailments than other areas of deprivation which influence well-being."[46] Positive changes in health care are however occurring (albeit slowly) in some Western countries. For example in Canada, increased consumer awareness and involvement in decision-making processes, facilitated by District Health Councils (DHCs)[47] have pressured service providers and administrators to take into account the holistic needs of those they serve.

SUMMARY

For Barbados, under the BLP, it cannot be denied that the documented health policy in terms of its ideology seems impressive for it gives the appearance of having the interests of all members of the community in its articulation, as verbalized by the following remark:

> Measures will be taken to ensure free and enlightened community participation, so that not withstanding the overall responsibility of the Government for the health

of its people as a whole, individuals and the community will assume greater responsibility for their own health and welfare, including self care. This participation is not only desirable, it is a social economic and technical necessity.[48]

The PRG policy, like that of the BLP, is impressive and inclusive. However, when compared to Barbados, the Grenadian system between 1979 to 1983 appears to be more holistic, with a focus on health promotion and education, and an emphasis on system coordination and linkage of health sector with other social and economic issues.[49] In order to ensure parity within the health care system, the PRG encouraged

the active participation of the public as a way of demystifying and democratizing the system of medicine and health care.[50]

A review of the provider perspective, however, shows that there is a mismatch between these declared policies and resource allocation and service delivery mechanisms. This is more evident in Barbados, during the 1979 to 1983 period, than in Grenada. In fact, by the BLP's own admission, the private/public dichotomy of the health care system produces a "disparity" in service delivery. From the interviews and discussions with the Barbadian and Grenadian providers it may be concluded that several PHC system elements are lacking in the models operating in their respective states. These deficiencies included:

1. A medical focus which inhibits the process of provider-user communication, program development based on actual needs, and service delivery that encompasses the WHO definition of health.
2. A lack of consistency in the way women were viewed and services were delivered to them as a group. This could stem from the lack of policy direction on gender issues.
3 A planning and decision-making process that largely excluded the involvement of working class women.
4. These weaknesses resulted in systems that were, for the most part, insensitive and inaccessible to working class women. Further analysis, however, is required to ascertain

whether working class women as a group are being deprived of basic primary health care and to determine the factors that may hinder access to services.

Notes

1. See Myra Buvunic et al (1979).
2. Interview, September 1992.
3. Interview, October 1992.
4. Ibid.
5. Interview, November, 1992.
6. Interview, October 1992.
7. Ibid.
8. Ibid.
9. Ibid.
10. Interview, September 1992.
11. Ibid.
12. Ibid.
13. Copperstock, Ruth, et al quoted by Agnes Miles. *Women, Health and Medicine:* 1991:161, see also Journal of Health Behavior (1977).
14. Rona Achilles "Beyond His and Her: Detecting Sexist Research in Health" *Health Promotion*, Special Issue on Women's Health.; Canada Health and Welfare 1987:9.
15. Ibid.
16. Connie Clement "Women and Health: From Passive to Active" *Health Promotion*, Special Issue on Women's Health.: Canada Health and Welfare Canada,1987:7.
17. Interview, September 1992.
18. Ibid.
19. See Jocelyn Massiah (1981); Pat Ellis (1986); and others.
20. Interview, November 1992 .
21. Interview, October 1992.
22. Interview, September 1992.
23. Ibid.
24. Ibid.
25. Ibid.
26. Ibid.
27. Ibid.
28. Interview, October 1992.
29. Ibid.
30. Interview, September 1992.
31. Dinesh Sinha (1988):132
32. Angela Briggs quoted by Jeanette Belle "Cultural Factors

Impacting on Women's Health": Unpublished Paper 1992:24; *see* also Grace Burke (1977); Mary Weinesse (1986) and others.

33. Interview, September 1992.
34. Interview, October 1992.
35. Ibid.
36. Ibid.
37. Development Plan 1988-1993 (Ministry of Health):29.
38. Interview, September 1992.
39. See Jocelyn Massiah (1981) and others.
40. See Peggy Antrobus (1991) and others.
41. Hilary Graham *Women Health and the Family* Great Britain: Harvester Press, 1984):83.
42. Interview, September 1992.
43. Ibid.
44. Mary Weinensee "Women's Health Perceptions in a Male Dominated Medical World" Diane K. Kiervik & Ida Martinson *Women in Health: Life Experiences and Crises* :W.B. Saunders Company 1986:19.
45. J. Richmond quoted by Mary Weinensee (1986):20.
46. C. H. Oelbaum quoted by Mary Weinensee (1986):20.
47. "A DHC is a local health planning board made up of concerned citizens who volunteer their time and expertise...They help plan health care services for their communities. DHCs are based on the belief that the people who live and work in a community are best able to determine their health needs." Quote taken from a pamphlet of the District Health Councils Partners in Health Planning.
48. Barbados Development Plan (1979 to 1983):139.
49. See James Ferguson (1990); Jules (1992).
50. Interview, October 1992.

CHAPTER 9

ASSESSMENT OF STATE
HEALTH CARE SYSTEMS IN
BARBADOS AND GRENADA:
THE WOMEN'S PERSPECTIVE

The previous chapter highlighted the strengths and weaknesses of the health care system of both countries as seen from the professional (provider's and administrator's) viewpoint. Of equal importance to the study is the consumer's (Barbadian and Grenadian women) perspective of the system's effectiveness, efficiency and sensitivity in meeting the needs of women. As such, a group of sixty working class women were given the opportunity to voice their opinions and concerns regarding service quality and delivery. Most of the Barbadian women were interviewed in September 1992. Some were interviewed in November 1992; all the Grenadian women were interviewed in October 1992.

CONDITIONS OF EXISTENCE

The following profile highlights the commonalities and differences in the lives of sixty working class women. The global picture presented of these women provides a more holistic view of the social, cultural, economic and political constraints that impact on their daily lives and consequently on their health and well-being. (See Appendix 3) The profiles are also significant in that they allow one to understand why working class women make choices, informed or uninformed, that may be ultimately beneficial or detrimental to their health.

Of the sixty women interviewed, twenty-seven or 45 percent were Barbadian and thirty-three or 55 percent were Grenadian women. Several parameters were used to establish the socio-economic status of the women: age, race, family status, family size, support systems/child care, educational attainment, employment status/job satisfaction, financial situation, housing conditions, transportation, religion, leisure time/relaxation and organization/group membership. The following gives a summary profile of the women interviewed. (*See Appendix 4 for a Detailed Demographic Profile of the Barbadian and Grenadian Women*)

Age

The Barbadian women interviewed were older than the Grenadian women. The average age of the Barbadian women was forty-four with the majority falling in the forty to fifty-nine age range, while the average age of the Grenadian women was thirty-seven, with the majority falling in the thirty to thirty-nine age range. This was not surprising since generally the Grenadian population is younger, with 46.6 percent of the total population falling between the age group fifteen to forty-four compared to 35 percent in Barbados.[1]

Race

Fifty-eight (96.7%) of the women were of African descent and only two (3.3%) were of Indian origin, one from each country. Again this is consistent with the ratio of Blacks to Indians in the general population. Barbados has a ratio of about 87.9 percent

Black to 0.8 percent Indian,[2] and Grenada has a ratio of approximately 84 percent Black and 3 percent Indian.[3]

Family Structure

Fifteen (55.6%) of the twenty-seven Barbadian women interviewed were married, four (14.8%) lived in common-law relationships, three (11.1%) were widowed and five (18.5%) were single. Only five (15.2%) of the Grenadian women were married, one (3.0%) lived in a common-law relationship, one (3.0%) woman was widowed and the other twenty-six (78.8%) were single. This striking disparity in the ratio of married to single women between the two countries is again consistent with the ratios in the general population, and may be attributed to the age differences and the tendency for people to marry at an older age. The 1980 Household Survey shows that 48.2 percent of Grenadian households were headed by single women.[4] Statistics show that approximately 42.9 percent of Barbadian households are female-headed.[5]

Number of Children/Family Size

The majority of Barbadian women (24 or 88.9%) had children. All but one of the married women had children; all three widowed women had children; two of the four women who lived in common-law relationships had children; and all five of the single women had children. Twenty-six or 78.8 percent of the Grenadian women had children. Twenty-two of the twenty-six who were single were mothers as were four of the married women. Neither the woman in the common-law relationship nor the woman who was a widow had children.

The Barbadian women generally had small families, consisting of one to three children; only one woman reported having five children. The small family size of the Barbadian women is consistent with that of the general population and may be attributed to the long established and successful government-assisted family planning program.[6] In contrast, the family sizes of the Grenadian women were generally large, ranging from two to eleven children; only one woman reported having one child. The larger populations in Grenada may be attributed to the lack of State-supported family planning.

Support Systems/Child Care

Both groups of women professed to having a wide variety of options to choose from should they need to talk about a concern or problem. The list included husbands, boyfriends, relatives, girlfriends and other friends, and God; the actual confidant selected depended on the nature and severity of the problem. For example, if the problem was a "woman problem," then girl-friends or doctors were consulted. Five of the Barbadian women, however confessed that they had difficulty in seeking advice or support from people and instead confided in God. One of the Grenadian women felt similarly and voiced her distrust for humans by stating, "I talk to God or myself. I can't tell everybody my business, they talk to others about you."[7]

For child care services, Barbadian women generally relied on older children and their mothers to look after the younger ones. Two of the women had children old enough to attend public nursery schools. The majority of the Grenadian women's children were of school age; only two needed care and this was provided by their grandmothers.

Educational Attainment

All of the Barbadian women interviewed received some level of formal training. All but one completed primary school, two reached Form IV level at secondary school and two had certification from polytechnic colleges, one in domestic science with a specialty in dressmaking and craft, and the other in secretarial studies. None of the women reported being involved in any continuing educational programs.

The two women who left secondary school early did so in order to contribute to the financial upkeep of their respective families. The following comments confirm this:

> I had to leave school at age thirteen because I come
> up the hard way. There were 5 children, my mother
> sent me to learn needlework. I didn't learn anything

much, the woman used to send me to pay all her bills.

I worked hard from the age thirteen. There were eleven children so I had to leave school and go to work. My first job was as an agricultural laborer.

In Grenada, although most of the women (31 or 93.9%) had formal schooling (two had no formal education at all), only about half of them completed primary school and only three of the women had reached secondary school (two left school at Form IV, age thirteen, due to financial difficulties; the other left after completing Form V). Two of the women who were denied a formal education stated:

I dropped out of school very early. I can't even remember the correct age, I think it was nine. I was always late because I had to look after the younger ones and some days I never got to go at all. I was always behind in the class and the other children made fun of me so I told my mother it was better if I stayed home and look after the younger ones. She was glad for the help so she agreed.

I had to leave school early. There was no money from anyone. My brother and I were abandoned by our mother, we lived with our grandmother. Our mother never came to look for us or helped and my father had his own life.

Again the difference in the educational levels between the Barbadian and Grenadian women is not surprising. Up to 1979, Barbados' literacy rate was 98 percent compared to Grenada's which was only 40 percent;[8] Barbados had developed mass education and literacy programs early[9] and had a highly-educated middle class. Although Grenadians in general recorded higher levels of people completing primary school (as the highest level of education attained) than Barbadians, a significantly larger percent of Barbadians went on to receive post secondary education than Grenadians and fewer were in the "no schooling" category. (See Table 9.1) The lack of, or limited, educational opportunities available to women, particularly working class women, has had a negative impact on them financially, since it has narrowed their employment opportunities.

Table 9.1
Barbados and Grenada: Percentage Distribution of Population Fifteen Years and Over* by Educational Attainment (Highest Level Attended) and Sex, 1980–82

Country	Sex	No Schooling	Primary (a)	Secondary (b)	Post-Secondary (c)	Others, Not Stated
Barbados	Female	0.6	53.0	39.9	2.0	4.5
	Male	0.5	50.1	40.9	3.8	4.7
Grenada	Female	1.8	81.6	14.7	0.6	1.3
	Male	1.5	83.1	12.2	1.8	1.4

*does not include those still attending school;

(a) includes infant school;

(b) includes all types of secondary/comprehensive, multi-tech and other secondary,

(c) includes university and other post-secondary.

Source: Sinha, Dinesh, Children of the Caribbean, 1945–1984 Progress in Child Survival, Its Determinants and Implications, 1988:89.

Employment Status, Occupation and Job Satisfaction

Only one of the Barbadian women reported being a full-time housewife; the majority worked in the service sector as restaurant workers, cleaners, cooks and domestics. The woman who had completed the domestic science certificate course was a primary school vocational teacher, while the other polytechnic graduate (the one with secretarial training) worked as a sales clerk. Three women were self-employed and operated home-based businesses: one was a dressmaker, one was a hairdresser and the other (one of the early school leavers) owned a catering business. The woman who owned the catering business had this to say about her experiences:

> I left school at age thirteen, but started working at age fifteen at a hotel washing wares and vegetables. I learned a lot and that is how I started my own business.

Similarly, the majority of the Grenadian women (21 or 63.6%)

also worked in the service industry in low-paying jobs as domestic, hotel and factory workers. Four of the domestic workers were from rural areas and augmented the family income by growing vegetables on family-owned land; their children or relatives would sell them in the market. Of the remaining five women who were employed, two were full-time farmers, one was a primary school teacher, one was a nurse and the other owned a small variety shop. The remaining seven women (21.2%) were unemployed. This unemployment rate is consistent with the 26 percent unemployment rate (1986 data) reported for the general Grenadian population.[10]

The women (Barbadian and Grenadian) who worked in the service industry reported changing their jobs a number of times. However, their lack of education and the availability of only low-skilled jobs confined their employment opportunities to similar areas of work and their choices for job advancement and enrichment were severely limited, a fact that was also true for most working class women in the general population.[11] Several of these women voiced dissatisfaction with their jobs and often found them to be stressful. They complained not only of the demands of the job, but also of the conditions under which they worked and the low compensation and limited perks they received. These grievances were expressed by two Barbadian women and one Grenadian woman.

Barbadian women:

> I worked from age 13 years. I used to work in the fields as an agricultural laborer. Then after I left that I worked in hotels but that was not easier. At least when I worked as a laborer I could get a piece of yam or eddo to take home; in the hotel you couldn't get a damn thing.

> The maid was laid off, the chef as well as the supervisor. That is kind of stressful because she wanted me to do my normal work as well as to do their work. Afterwards she brought in a chef, but I am still doing a lot of work.

Grenadian woman:

> I left school at age thirteen and had to do maid work. Sometimes it was very hard as the woman I worked for was not too nice. I am now a housekeeper at a guest house. Before this I worked as a maid at several hotels. My last job was very hard; I used to clean ten to twelve rooms from three to eleven p.m. at only twenty dollars a day.

In addition to their jobs, at which they all worked hard, the women had full responsibility in caring for their children and performing household and other family duties. These tasks added to their work load, reduced the time they had available for relaxation and contributed to the stress they were experiencing. Conditions that would certainly impact negatively on their health putting them at high risk for diabetes, high blood pressure and other chronic preventable diseases.

Financial Situation

Both the Barbadian and Grenadian women were struggling financially and reported that members of their family had suffered lay-offs and wage cuts. Their financial hardships reflect the economic times and shortages; in 1992 both Barbados and Grenada instituted Structural Adjustment Policies (SAPs).[12] These policies resulted in cutbacks in social programs which inevitably affected women's health.

As a result of their financial situation, many women resorted to buying only necessities such as food and were unable to meet the cost of school books, uniforms, bus fares and lunch money for their children. The Barbadian woman who had five children and worked as a domestic reported that things were particularly difficult for her and were getting worse.

> I am the only one earning and that is not much. The children's father never used to give them a lot of money but now it is even worse since he is laid off. Some days I don't want to get out of bed and face the same thing day after day. I just don't know what to do. I went to the welfare to try and get some help but that

was a waste of time because they don't have any money, yet they keep telling me to come back.

Similarly, the Grenadian women expressed difficulty; they all complained that they had insufficient money to buy food and pay rent. One woman, commenting on the present state of the economy, claimed that

> things have gone worse since 1983, a lot of people are not working, my husband got laid off several months ago now so we are living on the little money I make and that can't feed everybody.

The financial stress under which these women lived would have impacted not only on their health and well-being, but those of their children. The women were caught in a vicious cycle of poverty because of their lack of education, poor paying jobs and inadequate financial status.

Housing/Utilities

Only four (14.8%) of the Barbadian women owned their own homes, the other twenty-three (85.2%) rented. In contrast, twenty-six (78.8%) of the Grenadian women owned their own homes, although only fifteen (45.5%) owned both the house and the land; the others had built their homes on family-owned land. All twenty-seven Barbadian women had electricity and telephone services in their homes and all but one had piped water, indoor toilet and bath facilities. Five (15%) of the Grenadian women were without electricity, piped water and indoor toilet facilities, and only twelve (36.4%) had the use of a personal telephone. The others claimed that it was not difficult "to get a message" from a neighbor.

Religion

Only six (22.2%) of the twenty-seven Barbadian women interviewed claimed that religion played an important part in all aspects of their lives. These women identified themselves as being "Christians" and were either members of the Seventh Day Adventist Church or Jehovah Witness faith. Religion seemed to play an important part in the lives of all the Grenadian women and some of them claimed that "they started taking religion seriously after the revolution done." Although a majority of Grenadian women identified themselves as Roman Catholics, many attended the Testament Church of God where they found "companionship" with others. The increase in church going may have been to compensate for the sense of community and camaraderie and the clear leadership direction experienced during the PRG years when women's participation was encouraged.

Leisure Time/Relaxation

Very few of the women interviewed actually set aside time for themselves which could be termed "leisure" or "relaxation." Most of the activities counted as relaxation took place within their homes and included performing household activities such as cooking and sewing. Only four (12%) Grenadian women consciously took time out to go to the beach or for a swim, and only one Barbadian went to the beach, though infrequently and only when she felt like it. Very few of the Grenadian women either read or watched television; most of the Barbadian women watched the "soaps" on television. For those women who were religious, going to church was a popular form of relaxation and for the Grenadian women, in particular, so was gardening. The limited time available, and therefore allocated to leisure could be a result of the multiple roles women had as wager earners, home makers and care givers.

Organization and Group Membership

None of the Barbadian women interviewed belonged to, or participated in any social or autonomous women's organizations, other than the church. A number of the women felt that most organizations were linked to political parties and were not genuinely women's groups, in that they only dealt with "women at a certain level" and did not speak for "poor" women like themselves. One woman in particular related a feeling of alienation from the black middle class by stating that

Sometimes I feel inferior, they have the education I

don't. Some of them are doing something to help others but some who have certificates and get a big job and they have other Black people under them they treat you as dirt. They are the high-ups, they are the whites. They don't treat you as if you come from where they are.

This complaint of the lack of sensitivity shown by middle class women in the bureaucracy is not an isolated one. Education opportunities, social mobility and financial status have created a social distance between the Black middle class woman and her working class sisters.

Similarly, the Grenadian women were neither involved in nor were members of organizations, social or political, other than the church. A few of the women who came from St. George's (the capital city) reported that they had participated in community activities and women's groups during the revolution but had not done so since. Only two women who lived in rural communities claimed that they were still involved in community activities; however, they noted that the general level of participation was no longer as enthusiastic. One of them stated that participation

is not as strong as before, people are not coming out to meetings or giving support as they used to during the PRG days.

The sense of loss expressed by the Grenadian women exists because they remember the PRG days when they were involved and participated in the issues facing their country. Presently there are no such organizing forces: the NWO is no longer functional and the Women's Desk, which is under-financed and under-staffed lacks the ability to mobilize women. The effect of this has been the lack of coordination and direction with respect to addressing women's issues.

CRITIQUE OF THE HEALTH CARE SYSTEM

The ultimate goal of this study is to ascertain how state health policy and delivery systems impact on the lives and health of working class women in Barbados and Grenada. Accordingly, in order to effectively determine this, the perspective of women who utilize state health services (the polyclinics in Barbados and health centers/stations in Grenada) is paramount. To put their views and opinions in context and fully appreciate the health care system as a whole, the perspectives of women who use private clinics and services is also very important, since people who choose to pay for private health care often do so as a result of a previous negative experience or because of a particular perception about the state clinics.

Of the sixty women interviewed, forty-two always had used the state health clinics only (20 Barbadians, 22 Grenadians); six had previously used the state services but now only utilized private services (3 Barbadians, 3 Grenadian); eleven had always only used private services (5 Barbadians, 6 Grenadian); one Barbadian woman had previously used private services but now utilized public services; and two women exhibited no loyalty to either and utilized both at various times (1 Barbadians, 1 Grenadian).

During the interview process, the women who utilized the government clinics were asked to critique the state health care system. This included commentary on the overall quality of the system during the 1979 to 1983 period, and comparison of services delivered in that period with those they were presently receiving. The women who used the services of private doctors were asked to justify their choice. The women's statements were grouped under the following classifications:[13] service availability, service satisfaction, service accessibility and comparability to private health services. (*See Table 9.2 for Comparative Summary of Findings*)

1. SERVICE AVAILABILITY

• Human Resources
Both the Barbadian and Grenadian women complained about the lack of health care personnel in the state clinics. The current (1992) shortage in Grenada, however, seemed to be more acute and can be explained by the return/deportation of the Cuban doctors and other foreign health care personnel after the US invasion in 1983.

Doctors: From observation, there seemed to be a shortage of doctors in the Barbadian polyclinics in relationship to the number of patients seeking attention; this could be attributed to the low status and lack of incentive given to doctors working in PHC. The polyclinics are mainly staffed by junior doctors and non-Barbadian doctors. Sixteen (63.6%) of the twenty-three Grenadian women complained of shortages, stating that these did not exist during the PRG regime. Three of these women reflected on the situation:

> It was better. We had doctors, never mind they were Cubans, they were doing good.

> Now you can see a doctor but they are so few so you have to wait much longer than under the PRG.

> I had a baby under the PRG period and when I reach the hospital it was good I had no problems. It was definitely better then, there was always a doctor when you got to the hospital.

Nurses: The women also expressed concern about the shortage of nursing staff and the effect this had on the operations of the clinics and on them personally.

Barbadian women:

> The treatment is good, I use it whenever I am not feeling well. The only thing is the shortage of nurses, you have to wait a long time.

> I find the service has improved but the nurses still don't have time to talk to you.

Grenadian woman:

> During the PRG nurses used to come to the village where I live. Now I have to come to the clinic because the nurses have stopped coming.

Social Workers:

One Barbadian woman, in particular, felt that the services of social workers were needed at the polyclinics so that psycho-social problems and health-related issues could be dealt with. She reported that nurses were often too busy to talk to patients:

> The services here are okay, but the nurses are very busy. I think they should have social workers so you can talk to them if you have a problem. I never discussed this problem about my son's mental illness with anyone before today.

• Health Education/Preventive Services

The lack of health education sessions offered at the state clinics seemed to be an area of major concern for some of the women. The majority felt that only their presenting problem was addressed and not enough time was taken by either the nurses or doctors to explain some of their concerns (curative rather than preventive focus). As one Grenadian woman noted:

> The service is not too bad but they need to ask more questions and to do more examinations and to tell you more things about your health.

On the issue of health education, one Barbadian woman suggested that health concerns could be addressed while they were awaiting care:

> I feel the services are better now but I feel that while people are waiting they can be telling something, something about health, that way we won't feel bored waiting.

For the Grenadian women, there was also a general concern about the lack of preventative care delivered at the health centers in the post PRG period. One Grenadian woman, who worked in the area of pest control, expressed her frustration.

> I think at that time it was more serious than now because during the revolution I used to get a check-up three times a year. It is now October and this is the first one for the year. Last year I had it once and once again this year. In my job we are supposed to get a check-up every four months.

Another stated:

> I used to be able to get a pap smear every year or every two years but I haven't had one yet for the year.

• **Drug Services**
Several of the Grenadian women claimed that drugs were now (1992) in limited supply.[14] One woman described the current situation and expressed her opinion on the matter:

> Yes, the service has dropped since then [the revolution], medicine is very low. If you have a relative in hospital it is very rare that you will get the medication to help them. It has gone right down. They don't have this or that. I feel that a country should have good health care.

2. SERVICE SATISFACTION

• **Waiting Time**
Most of the women (Barbadian and Grenadian) complained of the long waiting periods endured during visits to the state health clinics. This particular service delivery problem seemed to be a consequence of the personnel shortages, especially at rural clinics. The Grenadian women reflected on this particular problem and generally agreed that the situation had gotten worse since 1983.

> The service is okay but I lose a whole day's work waiting. You have to wait too long.

> During the PRG days I never had to wait so long.

> Recently I took my daughter to the hospital, I had to wait a long time, but in the PRG days it was not like that.

> In order to see a doctor, you [now] have to give your name in advance for many days. I don't find that is good enough because if you get up in the morning and you sick as a poor person, you can't get medication

and it is very expensive.

The Barbadian women found their situation to be quite the opposite, conceding that there was a marked decrease in waiting time. They attributed this to the transfer of PHC services out of the hospital and into the polyclinics, and the introduction of an appointment system. One woman stated:

> The services are better now. Ten years ago when you came to the clinic you had a variety of people waiting for services, so you had to wait a long time. Now they have changed the system, it is more organized.

However, this is not to say that the waiting problem no longer existed, as these Barbadian woman attested:

> I know when I am coming here I have to lose a whole morning, but this is still better than before when you had to wait at the hospital for nearly a whole day.

> I always use the polyclinics but I find that I have to wait too long sometimes. Today, I have been here for over an hour already and I still don't have any idea when I'll see the doctor.

• Provider Attitudes

Doctors: Generally, the Barbadian women who used the state health services seemed satisfied with the polyclinic doctors. The Grenadian women, however, expressed some dissatisfaction with the current (1992) personnel, claiming that under the PRG doctors were far more accessible and had a more caring attitude. The Cuban doctors, in particular, were singled out for praise by all twenty-three of the Grenadian women who used the health centers/stations at one time or another. One woman shared this experience.

> The clinics were better then. We had better doctors and more doctors, so we did not have to wait for a long time. The Cuban doctors were very nice, they talked to you and attended to you like you were a person.

Nurses: Overall, the nurses were viewed positively by all the women (Barbadian and Grenadian) who used the state health clinics. Nurses were generally seen as "caring" and capable of providing reasonable service, despite the personnel shortages experienced at the clinics. The Barbadian women commented:

> It is a lot better organized than before and the nurses here are nicer than the ones at the hospital.

> The service is good, I have always used the polyclinics, the nurses I deal with are accommodating.

One Grenadian woman, who lived in a rural area, had this to say:

> I can't really complain, the nurses here are very nice, they encourage you, and give good advice.

• Sensitivity to Women's Health Issues

The majority of women (37.3% of the Barbadian women and 65.2% of the Grenadian) stated that they were either given inadequate information or no information at all with respect to health issues or concerns they had as women, and that not enough was being done generally in the area of women's health. A number of the responses by the Barbadian women highlighted the need for "woman-sensitive" health education:

> I feel some of the nurses and doctors in the polyclinics are not concerned enough. I feel we need more health information concerning women. Women's health is left out. At the clinics we get a lot of information about our children but not about us.

> I like coming to the clinic but I feel they should be telling us things that concern our health as women. I have four children but I feel I know very little about my body.

> I feel the nurses at the polyclinics are not pushy enough, everything is done very casually. I wasn't satisfied with the care.

When asked to clarify what she meant by "not being pushy enough," the woman who made the last comment explained that it was her first visit to the clinic and she had not been advised on pap smears or screening, or asked whether she was carrying out breast self-examinations. In general, the Barbadian women expressed a need for a special clinic for women which would provide them with information on areas of their health other than and in addition to family planning and maternal and child health information. One women who expressed this view stated:

> I don't think that the private doctors or government are meeting the needs of women. Right now we have to go to several different doctors. There is a need for a place where women can go for any kind of help not just health.

More Grenadian women complained about the lack of gender sensitive information and felt ignored/neglected since the invasion in 1983; 18.5 percent of them reported that several programs previously introduced by the PRG had been abandoned including health education classes, preventative services such as pap smear clinics, community meetings, and the milk program.[15] One woman stated:

> During the PRG they used to give milk but that is stopped now. You also used to get other things like eye check-up free.

• Quality of Care/Service
There were mixed sentiments about the quality of services offered by the state health clinics. Most of the Barbadian women were satisfied and had noticed improvements in the system since 1983. One Barbadian women confessed:

> [sometimes], I use another clinic, but I think health care in the polyclinic is generally good.

These Grenadian women also expressed satisfaction with the general quality of heath services:

> The service was good, it is about the same now.

> I am satisfied with the services now. There is a little drop in some areas, but generally it is the same.

> I like the clinic here, I get good advice for my children
> as well.

Others were dissatisfied with the quality of care and raised several concerns (18.5% of the Barbadian women and 86.9% of the Grenadian women). The Barbadian women felt that both doctors and nurses focused on presenting problems and did not try to find out the underlying cause. Some of the women expressed a need for a more personalized touch, complaining that the nurses were too busy to talk with them. However, most of the criticism was often leveled at the doctors.

> It is okay, but they can do a bit more. The last time I
> was here I came about my ear and the doctor just
> looked into my ear and prescribed medication, that
> was it.

> Well I find the service is longer, you have to wait and
> the examination is different because I haven't got one
> since I came here. I have asked the doctor for an
> examination but I didn't get any. I feel that I should
> have got one by now.

Twenty (86.0%) of the Grenadian women complained about the quality of care provided by the present state health centers, noting there had been significant deterioration. Although they attributed this to a number of other factors, the most consistent regarded the "lack of interest" shown by doctors as they carried out an examination and/or medical procedure. One Grenadian woman complained:

> I don't get the attention now that I used to get under
> the PRG.

• Information Sharing/Communication
All the women (Barbadian and Grenadian) complained that little information was made available to them by the clinic personnel. A criticism that is consistent with their comments regarding the lack of health education on key issues affecting their health. As one Barbadian woman simply put it:

> I don't find that they explain things enough.

• Infrastructure/Facilities

The Barbadian women were generally satisfied with the state facilities, as reflected in this woman's comments:

> The service is better than before and the buildings are nicer than before.

Their satisfaction stems from the fact that all the clinics in Barbados were either refurbished during the study period (1979 to 1983) or plans were set in place to build new ones.[16]

Several of the Grenadian women (52.1%), however complained about the poor physical conditions of the buildings in which the clinics were housed. Two women expressed their displeasure as follows:

> The clinics were better under the PRG, the government took steps to upgrade them so that when you went there you felt relaxed. The government was on our side from the head down.

> The clinics now are very run down and nobody comes to check on them. Before officials were always in the area checking on how things were going.

The women who used the major urban health stations were particularly annoyed with the excessive noise caused by private "mini-buses" which used the parking facilities immediately in front of the clinic. One woman was able to capture the sentiments of the others by stating:

> The buses have in front of the health center like a pig pen. I don't know how they expect people to come to this clinic. Sometimes you can't even hear yourself talking or what the nurse is saying. It is far too noisy. I think they should either move the clinic or the buses.

3. SERVICE ACCESSIBILITY

• Transportation

None of the Barbadian women identified transportation as a barrier to accessing health care services. This could be attributed to two factors: women generally attended the polyclinics located in their local parish; and Barbados has a good public transportation system. The availability and accessibility of public transport also allowed the women who used private health care services (usually located outside their areas of residence) to travel to the outskirts of Bridgetown (the capital), where a large percentage of the private doctors are located. In contrast, the Grenadian women did identify the lack of transportation as one of the primary barriers to accessing services. They claimed there was a shortage of state-owned transportation in certain areas and that the privately owned "mini-buses" mainly targeted the high density urban areas since these were considered more profitable.[17] Thus, women who lived in the rural areas experienced these difficulties to a greater degree. One woman claimed:

> None of the private buses come into this area. We have to walk out to the main road which is about 2-3 miles. During the PRG days the nurses used to come into the village so we didn't have to worry about going to the clinic. Now all that is gone so when I need to see a doctor I have to walk to the clinic which is very far away. I only come to the clinic when I am really sick.

Another Woman from Grenada stated:

> I have to come down to the clinic and there is no transportation where I live.

The rural women who used the services of private doctors were also faced with this problem since the majority of private services are based in St. George's (the capital). Inadequate transportation continues to affect access to health services.[18]

• **Finances**

One of the advantages of the state health care system in Barbados is that basic services are free, ensuring access to the economically disadvantaged. One woman lamented:

> I use it because I can't do any better. I would use a private doctor.

Grenada's payment policy was similar during the PRG regime; however the present NDC state health care is provided on a fee-for-service basis. The Grenadian women complained about paying for dental and other medical services which were all provided free by the PRG.[19] One of the women who suffered from diabetes categorically expressed her dissatisfaction with the situation.

> ....now I have to pay for my medication which is very expensive and sometimes it is not always available. During the PRG days I got everything free and I was able to get my medication right away. Now I sometimes have to wait 3-4 days.

Another woman expressed her frustration at having to pay for services that were once free.

> ....at that time,.... medicine was free. Now if you have cause to go to a private doctor you have to pay money as well as find more money to pay for the different medicines.

4. SERVICE COMPARABILITY TO PRIVATE HEALTH SERVICES

The seven Barbadian women and eleven Grenadian women who chose to use private health care services over the state's services, at one time or another, strongly defended their position, identifying several critical reasons for their decisions. Most of the women raised the issue of the long waiting times in the clinics. This was no surprise since almost all the women who used the state clinics had the same complaint. Of the six Barbadian women who only used the services of private practitioners (at the time of the study), four (66.6%) cited experiencing long waiting time was one of the reasons they no longer used the state health services. Two commented:

> When you go to the public clinics you not only have to wait a long time but are not treated well. There is always a long line of people waiting and waiting.

> When you go there you can't see a doctor, they always giving you an appointment to come back, and that time you may really be sick when they turn you away.

The women also raised a number of more specific concerns that question the credibility of state health services and thus require urgent attention. These included problems related to staffing and staff attitude; the amount of personal attention they received; the level of trust they had in the staff; the quality, reliability and continuity of care; and issues relating to class and religious/political persuasions, among others. One Barbadian woman summed up most of the concerns raised in the following assessment:

> I think polyclinic doctors to me are always in a hurry, they have so many people to look after. You can confide in your private doctor. If you want to discuss things with him. You can't do that with a polyclinic doctor. Today you can't say you will go back and see the same doctor next week. Your physician is always there for you and anything that I need I could call him. That is how I look at it.

As was done for the state clinic users, the comments and opinions of the private clinic users are categorized in grouping that surfaced inductively from their responses.

• Better Staffing at Private Clinics

Grenadian woman:

> I use a private doctor now but under the PRG I used the government services. We had more doctors and dentist based in Carriacou.

• More Favorable Provider Attitude/Personal Attention at Private Clinics

Barbadian women:

> My main reason is that I get better care and attention. I feel free to ask my doctor any question whatsoever, I feel free to ask my doctor anything and he has a caring attitude. I have gone to the polyclinics once or twice with my children, and they just seem to shuffle people in and out. They don't take time to find out

certain basic things whereas my doctor he takes time to find out; he could remember when I step in here I am Pam by name, he doesn't have to look up at my record to know who I am. He knows the various things that I complain for from time to time. He remembers when something pops again and he knows what was wrong with me years ago.

He can look back and see what he did then and how I reacted to the medicine and things like that.

You get personal attention, you can talk to him. At the polyclinics some of them don't even examine you. They write you a prescription without even waiting to hear from you, and then it is somebody else's turn to go in. My private doctor takes time to explain. You have to pay, but you are treated better.

He gave me a good examination and I can ask him questions. At the hospital they didn't have time to answer

Grenadian women:

I can talk to my doctor about problems and he explains everything

I have to wait at my private doctor but I still prefer coming here. You get personal attention.

Under the PRG I used to go to the public clinic. Health care was good then and we had several doctors. I changed because now there is only one government doctor and he has to see too many people.

• Lack of Confidentiality and Trust in State Agencies

Barbadian woman:

I prefer a private doctor. For example if you have a vaginal infection or some other problem that crop up for women you feel better going to a private doctor, because I don't trust the people at the polyclinics. The nurses tend to talk and things get out.

Grenadian woman:

The treatment is much better and less people know your business

• Poor Quality of Care at State Clinics

Barbadian woman:

At the polyclinics some of the doctors are always in a hurry. My private doctor takes time to explain. You have to pay but you are treated better.

Grenadian women:

I prefer the private doctor, when you go to the local government doctor you can't see them today. There is always some kind of problem. I find that when I or my children go to a private doctor and we need say an X-ray we get it quicker.

I started using a private doctor around 1985, because I was no longer satisfied with the treatment I got from the government clinic. Under the PRG I used the clinic, because it was good and it has several Cuban doctors, dentists and specialists who were either based in Carriacou or used to visit. At that time, all the services were free.

• Lack of Continuity in Care at State Clinics

Barbadian woman:

Every time I went to the hospital I saw a different doctor and when you think you are getting some help from one person then you see somebody else. The clinics are the same, you never get to see the same doctor.

• Classism Exhibited by State Clinic Staff

Barbadian woman:

> When you go to the public clinics, you are not treated
> well because you are poor. They make you sit there
> and wait nobody tells you anything. I have at least five
> doctors, including specialists. It saves a lot of time and
> thank you God until now I am able to pay for it.

• Political Persuasions

> One woman claimed that she used to take her children
> to the government clinics, but that she "never got
> involved with the PRG."

As illustrated the women who used private clinics were highly
critical of the state health clinics. In fact, most were so dissatisfied by services provided by these clinics that they went to great
lengths to obtain private services. Most of the Barbadian women
saved up in order to make these visits and some of them
"resorted" to the public clinics when they could not afford to pay.
One woman who was experiencing financial difficulties stated:

> I decided to join this clinic now since I can't afford to
> pay private fees.

Others who had established relationships with their doctors made
arrangements to pay in installments, and the few who absolutely
refused to use the polyclinics under any circumstances waited
until they could "afford it" to get a check-up. The women also
felt that "payment for service" was synonymous with good care
and prompt service. This caused one woman to state quite categorically,

> Sometimes I figure when you pay the money you get
> better treatment. I just feel if you don't have to pay
> maybe they just give you a hurry something. If you pay
> maybe they check you better.

The six women who claimed that they had always only used private doctors did so because they got a "thorough" examination
and their overall health and well-being was considered, in addition to the presenting medical problem.

SUMMARY

It may be concluded from the women's responses that health issues have not been approached in a holistic manner in either state under investigation. Presenting problems were/are treated without taking into account other health-related problems, gender specific issues facing women, and the socio-economic realities of their lives. Since most professionals (and some of the women) viewed health (women's health included) only in the context of the "absence of illness," they neglected to advise ongoing preventive care. This myopic perception of health was reflected in the few health education services available, and the limited exchange of information and communication that occurred between provider and client. Professionals either felt that women did not need and/or would not understand their conditions and therefore neglected to communicate relevant, user-friendly and sensitive information to them. Grenadian women, because of their community involvement and participation, were more likely to obtain health information and education from a number of sources. In contrast the Barbadian women lacked this empowerment and depended mainly on professionals, a top-down relationship characteristic of the traditional medical model of care. Most of the other complaints made by women using the state clinics were relatively minor in the sense that they were willing to deal with them if the primary health care issues of health education and prevention were taken care of. For example, one Barbadian woman stated that she would not mind waiting if the time was used more productively.

Women who reported seeking medical care from both private care and state health services seemed to be putting themselves at risk by over-utilizing treatments including medication from different sources. This dual approach to accessing services not only highlights the lack of continuity in care, but also the fragmentation and poor organization/management of the health care services.[20] This lack of coordination has encouraged poor accountability, information sharing, and lack of professional responsibility by practitioners, who although aware of this "shopping around" practice did little to address it. Further investigation of women who use private health care services (solely, or in combination with state health services) is needed since there seems to be an over-utilization of these paid services by women who are economically disadvantaged and can least afford it.[21] Those women who "saved" for their visits to private practitioners were, in particular, endangering their health. In situations like these, preventible conditions could rapidly deteriorate to severe acute or chronic levels and, thus, require long term treatment and care which is more costly.

From the interviews, it is quite apparent that the ideologies and political systems of the 1979 to 1983 states versus the post 1983 states influenced the delivery and quality of health services. The high political stability of Barbados and the ideological similarities of the BLP and DLP meant that the transition between these two governments in 1986 was relatively smooth and had little impact on the health care delivery system. As a result, the quality of services in Barbados remained consistent and little differentiation could be made by the women about services offered in the different time periods.

For Grenada, the situation differed drastically. Grenada was governed by parties that differed fundamentally in their ideological and political views. During the pre-study period, Grenada's health care system was largely underdeveloped. However, during the 1979 to 1983 period significant progress was made as the PRG began a process of "overhaul"' and "revitalization." Services were improved to a point where they compared with those delivered in other parts of the region, and in some cases (health education and community participation) were more advanced. For the Grenadian working class women, this period showed great improvements in their access to health care services. The gains were, however, reversed and services generally deteriorated after the invasion of 1983 and the return of a more conservative political thought. The change was, therefore, very noticeable, as was reflected in the women's highly comparative statements.

Table 9.2:
Critique of State Health Care by Barbadian and Grenadian Working Class Women: Comparative Summary Of Findings, 1979–1983 & Post 1983

*Researcher's observation and deduction

SYSTEM ELEMENTS	COUNTRY	1979–1983Period	Post 1983 Period
1. SERVICE AVAILABILITY			
• Human Resources:			
a) Doctors	Barbados	• Shortage experienced*	• Shortage still experienced
	Grenada	• Generally satisfied	• Shortage experienced
b) Nurses	Barbados	• Shortage experienced	• Shortage still experienced
	Grenada	• Generally satisfied; rural areas serviced	• Shortage experienced; rural areas not serviced
c) Social Workers	Barbados	Not mentioned	• Service needed
	Grenada	Not mentioned	Not mentioned
• Health Education & Prevention	Barbados	Not mentioned	• Services lacking/needed
	Grenada	• Some preventive services offered	• Situation deteriorated; few services previously offered, discontinued
• Drug Services	Barbados	Not mentioned	Not mentioned
	Grenada	• Generally satisfied	Medicines limited
2. SERVICE SATISFACTION			
• Waiting Time	Barbados	• Generally a problem; wait times too long	• Improvements seen
	Grenada	• Not considered a problem	• Wait times became too long

Table 9.2 Cont'd.
Critique of State Health Care by Barbadian and Grenadian Working Class Women:
Comparative Summary Of Findings, 1979–1983 & Post 1983

• Provider Attitudes:			
a) Doctors	Barbados	• Generally satisfied with doctors	• Level of satisfaction increased
	Grenada	• Generally satisfied with doctors (especially Cuban doctors)	• Some dissatisfaction expressed
b) Nurses	Barbados	• Particularly satisfied with nurses	• Level of satisfaction increased
	Grenada	• Level of satisfaction increased	• Still satisfied with nurses
• Sensitivity to Women's Health	Barbados	• Gender sensitive information/ services lacking	• Situation remained inadequate
	Grenada	• Few gender specific programs developed	• Situation deteriorated; few services previously offered, were discontinued
• Quality of Care/Service	Barbados	• Mixed sentiments: most satisfied	• Mixed sentiments: most satisfied and noticed improvements; major complaints: focus primarily on presenting problems, need for more personalized care
	Grenada	• Generally satisfied	• Mixed sentiments: most dissatisfied major complaint: provider's "lack of interest"

• Information & Communication	Barbados	• Generally lacking; one of the major complaints*	• Generally lacking; one of the major complaints*
	Grenada	• Generally lacking; one of the major complaints*	• Generally lacking; one of the major complaints*
• Infrastructure & Facilities	Barbados	• Generally satisfied	• Generally satisfied; improvements noted
	Grenada	• Generally satisfied	• Generally dissatisfied; deterioration noted
3. SERVICE ACCESSIBILITY			
• Transportation	Barbados	Not mentioned	Not mentioned
	Grenada	• Not a barrier to accessing services; services provided in rural areas	• Became a barrier to accessing services; adequate service no longer provided in rural areas
• Finances	Barbados	• Not a barrier to accessing services; state health services free (N.B. association of free state services with "poor people medicine"presented a barrier)*	• Not a barrier to accessing services; state health services free (N.B. association of free state services with "poor people medicine" presented a barrier)
	Grenada	• Not a barrier to accessing services; state health services free.	• Fee-for-service initiated; created an "unwelcomed" barrier to services

Key Reasons for not Using State Health Services (as stated by Private Users)

• Long wait times
• Poor staffing
• Lack of individualized/personalized care
• Lack of confidentiality and trust
• Poor quality of care and lack of continuity in care delivery
• Classism exhibited by staff
• Political persuasions

Notes

1. Norman A Graham, and Keith L Edward. *The Caribbean Basin to Year 2000 Demographic, Economic and Resource: Use Trends in Seventeen Countries.* :A West View Replica Edition, 1984:28.

2. Averille White "Profiles: Women in the Caribbean Project;" Social and Economic Studies. Vol. 35, No.2 :ISER, UWI June 1986:65.

3. Central Statistical Office (St George, Grenada, 1981).

4. Lenore Harney 1985:36.

5. Massiah, J " Women as Heads of Households in the Caribbean: Family Structure and Female Status." Paris: United Nations Educational, Scientific and Cultural Organization, 1983.

6. Byrne, J *Levels of Fertility in the Commonwealth Caribbean:1921-1965.* Kingston: ISER, UWI, 1972.

7. Interview, October, 1992.

8. Joseph, Rita "The significance of the Grenada Revolution to Women in Grenada." *Bulletin of Eastern Caribbean Affairs,* Vol. 7, No. 1: March/April, 1981.

9. See Stone 1986:129 and others.

10. Porter, 1981:91.

11. Gillings, 1987.

12. High external balance of payments forced Caribbean countries to institute SAPs Jamaica was the first to implement these policies, in 1977. Barbados, Grenada and Guyana implemented them in 1992. See Le Franc, 1990; Taylor, 1988.

13. Buvinic et al 1979.

14. Supported by Aberdeen, 1984 & others.

15. Supported by other reports See Harney 1985, Jules, 1992 and others.

16. See *Barbados Development Plan, 1983-1987*, Ministry of Health.

17. Confirmed by other reports, see Kaur, 1990:32.

18. Jules, 1992.

19. Supported by Aberdeen, 1984 and others.

20. See Alleyne, 1989.

21. See Le Franc, 1989.

SECTION 3:
BEYOND THE STUDY

Section Three of the study consists of a brief concluding chapter, which is sub-divided in three parts. Chapter 10 provides a summary of the theories that have been used by social scientists to analyze the state, generally, and in particular, the peripheral state. Special reference is also made to Barbados and Grenada and the effects of the State on women. The chapter also presents a snapshot view of health policy changes and/or reversals that occurred in both countries after the study period 1979 to 1983. These are used in combination with the detailed 1979 to 1983 analysis presented in Section 2, to produce a set of recommendations. The recommendations and future policy/service directions come from the women; the professional group and the researcher.

CHAPTER 10

CONCLUSION AND RECOMMENDATIONS

THEORIES ON THE STATE: A SUMMARY

There is no doubt that a theoretical understanding of the State, for example in terms of its assumption, concepts and principles of explanation, is critical for an appreciation of the countries isolated in the study. Although theories on the State in their most developed forms have been produced in advanced capitalist countries *(Chapter 1),* they have been useful for understanding the State in the periphery, given the role of the periphery in international capitalism.

Given that the conditions of women's lives constituted a fundamental part of this research, the views advanced by feminists in the advanced capitalist countries *(Chapter 1)* were also useful and therefore noted. It was, however, very evident that these capitalist State theories and their underlying premises were inadequate for explaining the *concrete* struggles of women within the two states. In analyzing the State in the periphery, and in particular Barbados and Grenada, it is essential to focus on their specific histories, their internal contradictions and struggles and the changes they have experienced.

While theories advanced by progressive Caribbean intellectuals *(Chapter 3)* were able to capitalize on these socio-historical experiences, they have been to a considerable degree produced by men and were therefore dominated by a number of "masculinist" assumptions. It is not the intention of this study to attack male scholars in terms of contributions and output since in many respects quality work was done. Nevertheless, their perspectives were flawed, essentially weak and in some instances irrelevant with respect to the experiences, struggles and conditions of women (who were the focus under consideration), since those issues of women's realities were mostly ignored.

Developments in Caribbean feminist theories *(Chapter 3)* represent an advance to the severely limited research done on some of the issues discussed in the study. Some interesting work is being done by Reddock (1984), Brereton (1988), Brodber-Wiltshire (1988), Green (1990), Carty (1991), Forde-Smith (1991), French (1991) and others, and needs to be acknowledged, supported and advanced upon. While these efforts need to be recognized (the work of Green deserves particular mention for its strong analysis), it is evident that there are still numerous gaps in the literature, and in a number of respects the literature remains highly underdeveloped. Efforts need to be intensified so that the marginalized strata of the society (working class women, the poor, unemployed and single-parents) can be examined more carefully and sensitively, in frameworks in which they constitute an essential part of the project.

The empirical data show that in Barbados significant progress and changes were made *(Chapters 6, 8 and 9)*, but what cannot be ignored is that Barbados essentially remained a neo-colonial state and reflected a number of associated weaknesses. The country never made any serious attempts to separate itself from external capitalist groups, and, consequently, molded itself into developing a "dependent capitalist" state, overly reliant on the West for its market, financial assistance, transport and tourism among other things. With respect to health, the programmes were also still externally directed (dependent), highly influenced by external capitalist institutions and policies (adapted British NHS model referred to and involved the U.S.-based Kellogg Foundation in its system evaluation), and severely restricted by the amount of outside financial assistance received (in total and the subsequent allocation made to health). Within Barbados itself, the specific class structure and the position of doctors (the most influential force in the health care system) within this class structure militated against any serious transformation of the health system.

> The medical profession in Barbados is very powerful, they are listened to certainly in our community; doctors and lawyers.... we are aware within the hospital environment that "consultants"are very powerful.[1]

Indeed, there were changes (National Drug Service, increase in the Polyclinics), but these changes (as in Grenada) have to be put within the framework of the country's development as a whole.

Grenada, as a peripheral state, suffered similar dependencies and associated problems *(Chapter 7, 8 and 9)*. While the country by 1979 (as a result of the revolution and the PRG gaining power) was no longer dependent on the West, it became dependent on other socialist (Cuba) regimes for its capital and human resources, and was influenced by the institutions and policies of these states (its PHC system was modeled after those in socialist China and other states). However, the PHC model appeared to suit the needs of the Grenadian general population (more so than the NHS model did the Barbadians) and contributed to improvements in the accessibility, equity and quality of health care delivered (through mechanisms such as the health care teams, the district nurses and the community health aides). While Grenada's experiment was indeed interesting and brought certain benefits to the working class, it also, like Barbados, had serious contradictions, particularly when examining the conditions of women. The women who saw improvements to their social and political status were essentially middle class/petit bourgeois and were not sufficiently connected to working women's lives. It may be argued that because the PRG was preoccupied with external threats, financial pressures, and hostility in an effort to defend the revolution many things were never dealt with or were left undone. This could have led to frustration and can be viewed as one failure of the revolution.

BARBADOS AND GRENADA IN THE POST-STUDY PERIOD:

POLICY CHANGES AND REVERSALS

There is no doubt that there is a shortage of human and financial resources and applied research within the region which confines the quality of work which is produced. However given the material that is available, a lot more could be done. Barbados is viewed in many parts of the Caribbean and the Western World as a model of progressive development but recent research seemed to be questioning the progress that the State claims to be making in a number of areas including health.[2] The system continues to be medically focused with emphasis in tertiary health care and little policy direction exists with respect to women's health.

The intervention in Grenada in 1983 resulted in severe setbacks not only structurally and programmatically, but it also affected the psychology of the people. Given their history of suffering under Gairy's dictatorship, the invasion of 1983 served to reproduce some of the insecurities, alienation and disempowerment that were evident during the Gairy era, and it may take a long time for the Grenadian people to develop a sense of confidence and identity that they seemed to display during the period under study (1979 to 83). However, the Grenadians have the advantage of experience and can be "revitalized" to address the identified gaps, especially and specifically as they relate to women.

FUTURE DIRECTIONS: RECOMMENDATIONS

The following recommendations include suggestions made by the health providers and women interviewed as well as the researcher's proposals for the delivery of timely, appropriate, comprehensive and quality services to working class women in Barbados and Grenada. These recommendations can also be extended to other women.

System Policy

- Governments must incorporate women's health into overall health policy development, taking into consideration the social and economic realities of women's lives.

- Governments must acknowledge the strong association between poverty and ill health and all state policy and programs that target low-income, single-headed households should reflect this relationship.

- Both countries need a more comprehensive and coordinated approach to the delivery of health care in order to respond to the various health care needs of women. Presently, inadequate attention is being paid to women's mental health, violence against women, and occupational and environmental health hazards.

- The development of health policy must be reflective of inter-sectoral cooperation which recognizes that "health" involves the concerted efforts of those inside and outside of the health sector.

- Women's groups and other voluntary organizations must be treated as equal partners, and collaboration with them in the development of policy, planning and providing of services to women must be ongoing.

- Reproductive health policy must be defined more broadly so that it integrates the total health of women over the whole life cycle and not just the child-bearing period.

Consumer/Community Participation

- Barbados should shift to a more community-based service which has true community involvement in the design and delivery service. Grenada should re-establish and build on the model of community participation used during the PRG tenure.

- Women must be consulted and involved in the creation and implementation of policies, programs and services related to their health and well-being.

Disease Prevention and Health Education/Promotion

• More attention or emphasis needs to be placed on preventive measures in the area of early detection, health education and treatment. Governments need to develop programs for women that deal with issues such as cancer control, diabetes control and education, blood pressure and obesity reduction, family violence prevention and control, sexually transmitted diseases and AIDS, nutrition and healthy life-styles.

• Governments need to institute worksite health promotion programs specifically designed for women .

• Organized breast-screening clinics and a centralized pap-screening program should be implemented by the State so that quality control measures and procedures are ensured.

Research/Training

• Education, clinical and emotional support services and research must be integral parts of program and project development.

• Governments should fund research which examines the sex-specific effects of environmental agents such as pesticides, chemicals and other toxic agents on the health of women.

• Gender sensitivity and awareness programs for health professionals must be part of their professional training as well as their continuing education so that the health implications of issues such as violence against women may be treated with priority.

More definitive courses of action cannot be prescribed without a comprehensive, holistic needs assessment that integrally involves working class women themselves. This is essential to the development of "internal" systemic structures which are supportive of and based on reality rather than perception (with respect to needs). Such undertakings require long term political and financial commitments, reallocation of power and control from the medical establishments to the community, and consumer empowerment and involvement; and must be done in a systematic, coordinated and integrated manner that encompasses all health and health-related sectors. A planning and coordinating body is needed to investigate the most effective and efficient means of achieving this and to oversee and monitor the process.

Although the study was conducted in Barbados and Grenada, the findings and recommendations may apply to other English-speaking Caribbean countries. Not only do they have similar historical experiences and socio-economic systems, but their health care systems and services have been developed along similar lines. However, one cannot and must not simply transplant the above recommendations made for Barbados and Grenada to other islands without engaging in a similar research of the state in question, making sure that the "voices" of working class women are heard and kept central within the review process.

Notes

1.   Interview, November 1992.
2 .   see Hilary Beckles (1990); Clive Thomas (1988).

BIBLIOGRAPHY

Caribbean Women

Antrobus, Peggy. "Women, Health and Development" for The Distinguished Lecturers Series, In Celebration of the Twenty-fifth Anniversary Of The Pan-American Health Organization (PAHO/WHO) Trinidad and Tobago, January 29, 1990.

Barrow, Christine "Anthropology, the Family and Women" *Gender in Caribbean Development*, (eds.), Patricia Mohammed & Catherine Shepherd:1988.

Cole, Joyce. "Official Ideology and the Education of Women in the English-speaking Caribbean 1835-1945" *Women in Education*, Vol. 5. ISER, University of the West Indies, Barbados: 1982.

Drayton, Kathleen. "Introduction to Joyce Cole, Ideology and the Education of Women in the English-speaking Caribbean 1835-1945" *Women in Education*, Vol. 5. Barbados: ISER, University of the West Indies: 1982.

French, Joan. *Hope and Disillusion: The CBI in Jamaica*, Association of Development Agencies (ADA), Jamaica: 1992.

Hodge, Merle. *Introductions to Perceptions of Caribbean Women*: ISER, 1984.

Massiah, Joycelin. Foreword to *Working Miracles: Women's Lives in the English-speaking Caribbean*, Cave Hill, Barbados: ISER, University of the West Indies, 1991.

Senior, Olive. *Working Miracles: Women's Lives in the English-speaking Caribbean*, Cave Hill, Barbados: ISER, University of the West Indies, 1991.

Articles
Government/Official Documents
West India Royal Commission Report. London: HM Stationery Office,
    June 1945.
General
McAfee, Kathy. *Storm Signals: Structural Adjustment and
    Development Alternatives in the Caribbean*: South End Press,
    1991.

Health
Alleyne, George A. O. "Health and Development in the Caribbean
    Perspectives," Seventh Eric Williams Memorial Lecture. Port-of-
    Spain, Trinidad and Tobago: April 15,1989.

GRENADA

Books
Ambursley, Fitzroy & Dunkerley, James. *Grenada Whose Freedom?*
    London: Latin American Bureau, 1984.
Ambursely, Fitzroy & Robin Cohen. (eds.). *Crisis in the Caribbean*.
    New York: Monthly Review Press, 1983.
Ambursley, Fitzroy. *The Grenadian Revolution-1983: The Political
    Economy of An Attempt at Revolutionary Transformation in a
    Caribbean Mini-State*. University of Warwick: Ph.D. dissertation,
    1985.
Bishop, Maurice. *Forward Ever: Three Years of the Grenadian
    Revolution.*. Sydney, Australia: Pathfinder Press.
Brizan, George. *Grenada Island of Conflict: From Amerindians to
    Peoples' Revolution 1498 to 1979*. London: Zed Press, 1979.
Emmanuel, Patrick; Farley Braithwaite; & Udine Barriteau. "Political
    Change and Public Opinion in Grenada 1979 to 1984."
    Barbados: University of the West Indies, ISER Occasional Paper
    No. 19, 1986.
Ferguson, James. *Grenada Revolution in Reverse*. London: Latin
    American Bureau, 1990.
Ferguson, James. *Far From Paradise: An Introduction to Caribbean
    Development*: 1990
Gonsalves, Ralph. *The Non-Capitalist Path to Development; Africa &
    The Caribbean*. London: 1981.
Heine, Jorge. *A Revolution Aborted: The Lessons of Grenada*.
    Pittsburgh, University of Pittsburgh.
Jules, Didacus & Rojas, Don. (eds.). *Maurice Bishop: Selected
    Speeches 1979 to 1981*. Cuba: Casa de Las Americas, 1982.
Lewis, Gordon. *Grenada: The Jewel Despoiled*. Baltimore: John
    Hopkins University Press, 1987.

Marable, Manning. *African & Caribbean Politics: From Kwame Nkrumah to Maurice Bishop.* London: Verso, 1987.

O. Shaughnessy, Hugh. *Grenada: Revolution, Invasion and the Aftermath.* London: Sphere Books, 1984.

Payne, Anthony, Paul Sutton & Tony Thorndike. *Grenada: Revolution and Invasion.*: 1984.

Pryor, Frederic. *Revolutionary Grenada: Study in Political Economy.* New York: Praeger, 1986.

Sandiford Gregory & Vigilante Richard. *Grenada: The Untold Story.* London: Madison Books, 1984.

Searle, Chris (ed.). *In Nobody's Backyard, Maurice Bishop's Speeches 1979 to 1983: A Memorial Volume.* London: Zed Press, 1984.

Stone, Carl. *Power in the Caribbean Basin: A Comparative Study of Political Economy.* Inter-American Politics Series, 1986.

Sunshine, Kathy. *Grenada, The Peaceful Revolution.* Washington: EPICA, 1992.

————. *Death of a Revolution.*

Ministry of Health Publications

Nurse Cortez & Dr. Clarke, George. "Three Year Health Plan 1982-1985." (Draft) Grenada, Carriacou & Petit Martinique: Ministry of Health, 1982.

Other Government & Party Publications

Bishop, Maurice. Address by Prime Minister of Grenada at the Bloody Sunday Rally at Seamoon. St. Andrew's : November 16, 1980.

————. "Fight Unemployment Through Production." Speech by Cde. Prime Minister of Grenada to Conference on Unemployment. The Dome, Grand Anse: Grenada Fedon Publishers, 1982.

Coard, Bernard. Minister of Finance & Planning, Peoples Revolutionary Government. Report of the National Economy for 1981 and the Prospects for 1982.

The 1973 Manifesto of the New Jewel Movement.

Articles

Alleyne, Candia. "Changing Perspectives on Health Care Development in Grenada." Bulletin of Eastern Caribbean Affairs 7, No. 1: March-April, 1981.

Bishop, Maurice. "Revolution in Grenada: An Interview with Maurice Bishop." Black Scholar: January-February, 1980.

Davis, Lewis A. *Reform and Revolution in Grenada 1950 to 1981.* Cuba: Casa De las Americas, 1984.

De Riggs, Chris. "Health Care: Achievements and Prospects." *Grenada is not Alone*: Speeches by the PRG at the first International Conference in Solidarity with Grenada. St George's : November

Fedon Publishers, 1981.

Joseph, Rita. "The Significance of the Grenada Revolution to Women in Grenada" Bulletin of Eastern Caribbean Affairs, Special Issue, 7, No. 1: March-April, 1981.

LaGuerre, John. "Future of Democracy in Grenada" Caribbean Affairs Vol. 1 No. 3: July-September, 1988.

Lowther, William. "Caribbean Coup: Revolt in Reggae Time." Frontlines, Macleans: April 9, 1979.

Mandle, Jay. *Big Revolution, Small Country, The Rise and Fall of the Grenadian Revolution*. The North-South Publishing Co., 1985.

Naipaul, V.S. "An Island Betrayed: Grenada Revolution/Coup 1979." Harper's Magazine: 1984.

Ryan, Selwyn. "The Grenada Questions: A Revolutionary Balance Sheet." Caribbean Review 13 (Summer): 1984, 6-9.

Wilkson, Audine. "A Select Bibliography." Bulletin of Eastern Caribbean Affairs 7, No.1: March-April, 1981.

Newspapers

The Free West Indian. Address by Prime Minister Maurice Bishop on Primary Health Care in the Parish of St. David's: October 24, 1981:5.

The Trinidad and Tobago Review : June, 1979: 6."Grenada Special: Grenada revolution: A major setback for regional unity." Insights: 1979.

Anne Walker. "Grenada's Women, Four Years after March 1979."The Caribbean Contact. Barbados: February, 1983.

Non-Print Sources (including coded interviews)

Pamphlets

Festival of Women: International Women's Year 1975, "Grenada Relies on Women."

Unpublished Sources

Jules, Didacus. Education and Social Transformation in Grenada 1979 to 1983. Ph.D. Thesis. Madison: The University of Wisconsin, 1992.

Porter, Rosemary Anne. Women and the State: Women's movements in Grenada and Their Role in the Grenadian Revolution 1979 to 1983. Ph.D. Thesis, Temple University; 1986.

Williams, Dessima. Achieving Sovereignty Under Hegemony: US-Grenada Relations 1979 to 1983. Ph.D. dissertation. Washington, DC: American University: 1992.

BARBADOS
Books

Beckles, Hilary. *A History of Barbados from Amerindian Settlement to Nation State*. Cambridge University: 1990.

Cumper, G.E (ed.). *The Economy of the West Indies*. Jamaica: ISER, University of the West Indies, Jamaica: 1960.

Dann, Graham. *The Quality of Life in Barbados*. Macmillian Publishers, 1984.

Fields, Gary S. "Growth, Employment, Inequality and Poverty in Trinidad, Barbados & Jamaica." Working Paper No. 41, Department of Economics, Cornell University, December, 1981.

Vallen, Jacques & Lorez, Alan D. (eds.). *Health Policy, Social Policy and Mortality Prospects*: International Union for the Scientific Study of Population (IUSSP), 1985.

Worrell, DeLisle. (ed.). *The Economy of Barbados 1946 to 1980*: Central Bank of Barbados, 1982.*Ministry of Health Publications.*

Annual Reports of the Chief Medical Officer of Health: 1979, 1983, 1984 and 1987-88.

Final Technical Report, "A Study to Evaluate the Quality of Care Provided to Women and Children at Polyclinics in Barbados." Population Council in collaboration with the Ministry of Health, Barbados and Women and Development Unit (WAND), UWI, July 1990.

Other Government & Party Publications

"Barbados Development 1979 to 1983, Planning for Growth." Ministry of Finance & Planning: Barbados, Government Headquarters.

Barbados Development Bank 11th Annual Report 1979 to 1980.

Financial Statement & Budgetary Proposal, April 1979.

"Where Are We Now? An Assessment Of The Status Of Women In Barbados." Bureau of Women's Affairs, Ministry of Labor and Community Development, 1985.

House of Assembly Debates (Official Reports) Second Session: 1976 to 1981.

Labor Market Information Report 1976 to 1983: Ministry of Labor, Social Security and Sport, September 1984.

The Report of the National Commission on the Status of Women in Barbados, Volume 1 & 2: May 1978.

Articles

Forde, Norma Monica. "The Status of Women in Barbados: What Has Been Done Since 1978." Occasional Paper No. 5. Eastern Caribbean, UWI, Cave Hill Campus, Barbados: ISER, 1978.

Newspapers

"Barbados: No Early Recovery." Advocate News:August 1982:16.

"Barbados Health Care Praised; Sir Kenneth Hunte." Advocate News: Saturday 17 December, 1983:1.

"Emergency Powers Now in Barbados." Caribbean Contact: June 1982: 16.

Caribbean Contact, August 1, 1982.

"Adams: Barbados and the Caribbean." The Caribbean Chronicle: 1981.

The Nation, October, 1983:7.

Non-Print Sources
Pamphlets

Unpublished Sources

Bell, Jeanette "Cultural Factors Impacting on Women's Health." Barbados:WAND, 1992

1.The State in Advanced Capitalist Societies

Babbio, M. *"Is there a Marxist Theory of the State?"* Telos 35: Spring, 1978:5 -16.

Baran, P. *The Political Economy of Growth.* : Monthly Review Press, 1957.

Block, Fred. "Contradictions of Capitalism as a World System" *Insurgent Sociologist.* Eugene, Oregon USA: Winter, Vol. 1, No. 2, 1975.

Braverman, Harry. *Labor and Monopoly Capitalism: The Degradation of Work in the Twentieth Century.* Monthly Review Press, 1974.

Cockbourn, C. *The Local State.* London: Pluto Press, 1977 Ch. 6.

Collier, David. (ed.) *The New Authoritarianism in Latin America:* Princeton University Press, 1979.

Currie, H Mac L. *The Individual and the State,.* The Ancient World: Source Books, Aldine Press, 1973.

Dale, Roger. *The State and Educational Policy.* Toronto: OISE Press, 1989.

Draper, Hal. *Karl Marx Theory of the Revolution.* New York: 1977, Part 1, Books 1 & 2.

Engels, Frederick. *The Origins of the Family, Private Property and the State*, Introduction by Eleanor Burke Leacock. New York: International Publication, 1990.

Evans, Peter E. et al. (ed.). *Bringing the State Back In*: Cambridge University Press, 1985.

Gramsci, Antonio. *Letters from Prison*, (ed.). Lynne Lawner: The Noonday Press, 1973.

James, C.L.R. "State Capitalism and World Revolution" *Facing Reality*. Detroit: 1969.

Jessop, B. "The Capitalist State." Cambridge Journal of Economics: 1977.

——. *State Theory*. : Polity Press, 1990:338.

Lenin, V. I. "Report on the National and Colonial Question." *Selected Works in Three Volumes*. Moscow: Progress Publishers, 1971, Vol.3.

London Edinburgh Weekend Return Group. *In and Against the State*: Pluto Press, 1980.

Mandell, Ernest. *Late Capitalism*. London: New Left Books, 1975.

Marx, Karl. *Capital*: Lawerence & Wishart, 1974, Volume 1.

Marx, K. and Engels, F. *Selected Works* :Lawerence & Wishart, 1986.

Miliband, R. *The State in Capitalist Society*. London: Weidenfield and Nicolson, 1968.

——. "State Power and Class Interest." Monthly Review: 1983 No. 138, pp. 37-68.

——. "The Capitalist State. Reply to Poulantz." New Left Review: 1970, No. 59. pp. 53-60.

Offe, C. "The Theory of the Capitalist State and the Problem of Policy Formation." *The State and Contradiction in Modern Capitalism*, (ed.). L. Linberg et al., Lexington, Mass: 1972.

Ollman, Bertell. "Theses on the Capitalist State." Monthly Review: 1982, Vol. 34, No. 7, p.40.

Open University. *Politics, Legitimacy and the State*. London: Open University Press, Units 14 and 15, p.9-10.

Poulantaz, Nicos. "The Problem of the Capitalist State." New Left Review: 1969, No. 58, pp. 67-78.

——. "Political Power and Social Classes." New Left Review. London: 1973.

——. "The Capitalist State: A Reply to Miliband and Laclau." New Left Review: 1976.

2. State Formation in the Periphery/Caribbean

Ahmad, G. "The Neo-Fascist State": Notes on the Pathology of Power in the Third World. *International Foundation for Development Alternatives*: 1980, Sept-Oct., 19:15-26.

Ake, Claude. "The Congruence of Political Economies and Ideologies in Africa" Peter C.W. Gutkind and Immanuel Wallerstein. (eds.) *The Political Economy of Contemporary Africa*. Beverly Hills, London: Sage, 1976.

Alavi, Hamza. "The State in Post-Colonial Societies: Pakistan and Bangladesh." *New Left Review* 74: July/Aug , 1972, 54 - 81.

——. *"Sociology of Developing Societies"* (ed.). Monthly Review Press: 1972.

Amin, Samir. *Class and Nation*: Historically and in the Current Crisis. New York and London: 1980.

Andaiye. "Women in Political Parties." *Caribbean Contact*. Barbados: Caribbean Conferences of Churches, 1988.

Ambursely, Fitzroy. "Grenada: The New Jewel Movement." Fitzroy Ambursely & Robin Cohen (eds.) *Crisis in the Caribbean* :1983, 9:191.

Ambursely, F. and Cohen, R. *Crisis in the Caribbean*, NewYork and London: 1984.

Aziz, Sartay. "The World Food Situation and Collective Self-Reliance." *World Development*: Oxford, May-July, 1977, Vol.5, Nos. 5-7.

Baghu, Amiya Kumar. *The Political Economy of Underdevelopment*.: Cambridge University Press, 1982.

Beckford, George L. et al. *A Caribbean Reader on Development*. Jamaica: FES, 1986.

Campbell, H. "The Commandist State in Uganda." University of Sussex, England: Political Studies Research in Progress Seminar Paper, April, 1977.

Craig, Susan. *Contemporary Caribbean Sociological Reader*. Trinidad and Tobago : 1982, Vol. 12.

Collier, David.(ed.). *The New Authoritarianism in Latin America*: Princeton University Press, 1979.

Deere, Carmen Diana et al. *In the Shadows of the Sun*. Caribbean Development and U.S. Policy, A PACCA Book: Westview Press, 1990.

Dos Santos, Theotonio. "Socialism and Fascism in Latin America Today."

The Insurgent Sociologist. Eugene, Oregon, USA: Fall, 1977, Vol. VII, No. 4.

Emmanuel, Patrick. *The Role of the State in the Commonwealth Caribbean*, Working Paper No. 38, Jamaica: ISER, 1990.

Frank, Andre Gunder. *Crisis: in the Third World*. London: Heineman, 1981.

——. *"Capitalism and Underdevelopment in Latin America."* Monthly Review. New York: 1967.

Girvan, N. et al. "The IMF and the Third World: the Case of Jamaica, 1974-1980." *Development Dialogue* : 1980, Vol. 2, pp. 113-155.

Gonsalves, R. "The Non-Capitalist Path to Development.": 1981.

Goulbourne, Harry. *"The Problem of the State in Backward Capitalist Societies."* Africa Development: 1981, Vol. 34 V!, No. 1 pp. 45-70.

——. (ed.). *Politics and State in the Third World*. London: 1978.

Harris, Donald J. Notes on the question of a national minimum wage for Jamaica in *Essay on Power and Change in Jamaica*. (eds.) C.

Stone and A. Brown: Jamaica Publishing House, 1977, 9:157-167.

Hein, Wolfgang & Steinzel Koniod. "*The Capitalist State and Underdevelopment in Latin America*: The Case Of Venezuela." Kapitalistate 2: 1973.

Lewis, Gordon K. *The Growth of the Modern West Indies.* : London, MacGibbon & Kee, 1968.

——. *Main Currents in Caribbean Thought*: The Historical Evolution of Caribbean Society in its Ideological Aspects 1492-1900: John Hopkins University Press, 1983.

Lewis, W. Arthur. *The Industrialization of the British West Indies,* Barbados: Reprint, Government Printing Office, 1950.

——. *Labor in the West Indies*: the Birth of a Workers' Movement. London: New Beacon Publishers, 1977.

Less, Colin. "*The Overdeveloped Post-Colonial State*: A Revelation." Review of African Political Economy: Jan-April, 1976, No. 5, pp. 39-48.

Mamdani, Mahmood. "*Politics and Class Formation in Uganda.*" New York: Monthly Review Press, 1976..

Manley, M. *Jamaica: Struggle in the Periphery.* London: Third World Media Ltd., 1982.

Manigot, A. P. "The Difficult Path to Socialism in the Caribbean." Richard Fagan (ed.) *Capitalism and the State in U.S. and Latin American Relations*: Stanford University Press, 1979.

Morrissey, Marietta. "*Towards a Theory of West Indian Economic Development.*" Latin American Perspective: Winter, 1981, Issue 28, Vol. V111, No.1.

Nanton, Philip. "The Changing Patterns of State Control in St. Vincent and the Grenadines." Fitzroy Ambursely and Robin Cohen (eds.) *Crisis in the Caribbesn*: Monthly Review Press, 1983, 10:223.

Ottman, H. *The Tanzanian State:* Monthly Review Press 26, Dec., 1974: 46-57.

Reddock, Rhoda."Women, Labor and Struggle in Twentieth Century Trinidad and Tobago." Doctoral dissertation, University of Amsterdam.:1984.

Riverie, Bill. *State Systems in the Eastern Caribbean:Historical and Contemporary Features.* Jamaica: ISER, 1990.

Rodney, Walter. *How Europe Underdeveloped Africa.* Howard University Press, 1974.

Saul, John. "*The State in Post-Colonial Societies: Tanzania.*": Socialist Register, 1974.

——. *State and Revolution in East Africa.* NewYork and London: 1979.

Shivji, Issa. *Class Struggles in Tanzania.* NewYork and London: 1976.

——. "State and Constitution in Africa: A New Democratic

Perspective." *International Journal of the Sociology of Law* : 1990, Vol. 34 18, No. 4, p 383.

Stone, C. *Decolonization and the Caribbean State System: The Case of Jamaica.* New York: Center for Inter-American Relations, 1978.

Thomas, Clive. *The Rise of the Authoritarian State in Peripheral Societies.*: Monthly Review Press, 1984.

———. "The Non-Capitalist Path as Theory and Practice of the Colonization and Socialist Transformation." *Latin American Perspectives.*: 1987 Vol. 5, No. 2, pp. 10-28.

Williams, Eric. *From Columbus to Castro: The History of the Caribbean 1494 to 1969.* :Andre Deutsch, 1970.

3. Feminist Perspectives on the State

Andrew, Caroline. "Women and the Welfare State." *Canadian Journal of Political Science* XV11: 4, December, 1984.

Armstrong, Pat & Armstrong, Hugh. *Theorizing Women's Work.*: Toronto, Garamound Press, 1990.

———. *The New Practical Guide to Canadian Political Economy.*:Toronto, James Lorimer Company, 1985.

———. "Political Economy and the Household: Rejecting Separate Spheres." *Studies in Political Economy*, 17: Summer, 1985:167-177.

Barrett, Michele. *Women's Oppression Today.*: London, Verso Books, 1980.

Bulbeck, Chilla. *One World, Women's Movements.*: London, Pluto Press, 1988.

Burstyn, Varda & Smith, Dorothy. *Women, Class, Family and the State.*: Canada, Garamound Press, 1984.

Caranagé, Charlene. *Double Day, Double Bind: Women Garment Workers.*:The Women's Press, 1984.

Carty, Linda & Brand, Dionne. "Visible Minority Women - A Creation of the Canadian State: Feminist Perspectives on the Canadian State.": Toronto: *Resources for Feminist Research*, OISE, September, 1988, Vol.17, No.3.

Chapman, Tom & Cook, Juliet. "Marginality, Youth and Government Policy in the 1980s." *Critical Social Policy*, : Summer, 1988, Issue 22, Vol. 8 No. 1.

Davis, Angela. *Women, Race and Class*, New York: Random House, 1980.

———. (1990) *Women, Culture and Politics.*:Vintage Books, 1990.

Dahlekrup, Drude. "Confusing Concepts, Confusing Reality: a Theoretical Discussion of the Patriarchal State." Anne S. Sassoon (ed.) *Women and the State.* London: Hutchinson, 1987.

Fatton, Robert. "Gender, Class and State in Africa." Staudt & Parpart (eds.) *Women and the State in Africa* :1990, Chap. 3.

hooks, bell. *Black Women and Feminism*: Ain't I A Woman: Smith End Press, 1981.

Hull, Gloria T, et al. (eds.) *But Some Of Us Are Brave: Black Women's Studies.*: New York, The Feminist Press, 1982.

Jacobs, Susan. "Zimbabwe: State, Class and Gendered Models of Land Resettlement." Staudt & Parpart (eds.) *Women and the State in Africa* : Boulder & London, 1990.

MacKinnon, Catharine A. "Feminism, Marxism, Method and the State." :Yale University Press, 1987.

———. *Feminism, Unmodified: Discourses on Life and Law.*: Harvard University Press, 1987.

———. *Toward a Feminist Theory of the State.*: Harvard University Press, 1989.

Mohanthy, Chandra Talpade, et al. *Third World Women and the Politics of Feminism.*: Indiana University Press, 1991.

Mies, Maria. *Patriarchy and Accumulation on a World Scale: Women in the International Division of Labor.*: Zed Books Ltd., 1986.

———. *Women the Last Colony.* : Zed Press, 1988.

Mitchell, J. & Oakley, A. *What is Feminism?* Oxford: Blackwell, 1988.

Molyneux, Maxine. "State Policies and the Position of Women Workers in the Peoples' Democratic Republic of Yemen 1964-77." *Women and Development 3.* Geneva: International Labor Office, 1984.

Ng, Roxanna. Introduction in *Women, Class, Family and the State* by Burstyn, Varda & Smith, Dorothy E.: Toronto, Garamound Press 1985.

Oakley, A. *The Sociology of Housework.* : Oxford, Martin Robertson, 1994.

Ramazanoghu, Caroline. *Feminism and the Contradictions of Oppression.*: London and New York, Routledge, 1989.

Randall, Melanie. "Feminism and the State: Questions for Theory and Practice." *Resources for Feminist Research* , OISE, 1988, 17:10-16.

Rowbothan, Shelia. *Women, Resistance and Revolution.* : Penguin Books Ltd, 1972, Chap.3.

Smith, Dorothy E. *Feminism and Marxism.* Vancouver: New Star Books, 1977.

Staudt, Kathleen A. & Parpart Jane L. (eds.) *Women and the State in Africa.* :Boulder & London, Lynne Reinner Publishers, 1990.

UNIFEM Occasional Papers 10. "Preliminary Assessment of the Impact of Stabilization and Structural Adjustment Program on Selected UNIFEM Programs and Supported Projects." New York: UNIFEM, Jan., 1990.

Wireringa, Saskia. (ed). *Women's Struggles and Strategies*. Aldershot, England: Gower, 1988.

4. Women and Health

Arber, S., Gilbert, G.N. and Dale, A. "Paid Employment and Women's Health: a Benefit or a Source of Role Strain?" *Sociology of Health and Illness*. :1985, 7(3) 375-400.

Barta, David H. and Thacker Stephen B. "Policies Towards Medical Technology: A Case of Electronic Fetal Monitoring." *American Journal of Public Health*.:1979: 69, No.9, 931-35.

Blaxter, M. and Patterson, E. *Mothers and Daughters: A Three Generational Study of Atti tudes and Behavior*. London: Heinemann, 1982.

Burnell, I. and Wandsworth, M. *Children in One Parent Families*.: University of Bristol, Child Research Unit, 1981.

Cottingham, Jane. "Women and Health." *Women and Development: A Resource Guide*. :ISIS, 1984, p.143-157.

Cutrufelli, Maria Rosa. *Women of Africa: Roots of Oppression*. London: Zed Press, 1983.

Doyal, Lesley. "Women Health and the Sexual Division of Labor." *Critical Social Policy*. : Summer, 1983, No.7, 21-23.

——. *The Political Economy of Health*. Boston: South End Press, 1981.

Director-General, WHO. *Women, Health and Development*. Geneva: WHO Offset Publication, 1985.

Ehrenrich, Barbara & English, Deirdre. *Witches, Midwives and Nurses: A History of Women's Healers*. Old Westbury, New York : Feminist Press, 1972.

Fendall, N.R.E. "Primary Medical Care in Developing Countries." *International Journal of Health Services*. : 1972, Vol. 2, No. 2, p.304.

Graham, Hilary. *Women, Health and the Family*. Great Britain: Harvester Press, 1984.

Gordon, Linda. *Women's Body, Women's Rights: A Social History of Birth Control in America*. New York: Grossman, 1976.

Kjervik, Diane K., & Martinson, Ida M. *Women in Health and Illness: Life Experiences and Crises*.: W.B. Saunders & Company, 1987.

Hartman, Betsy. *Reproductive Rights and Wrongs: the Global Politics of Population Control and Contraceptive Choice*. New York: Harper and Row, 1987.

Hibbard, Judith H. and Clyde R. Pope. "Women's Roles Interest in Health and Health Behavior." *Women and Health*. :1987, Vol. 2.

Ibrahim, M.A. "The Changing Health State of Women." American

Journal of Public Health. : 1980 Vol. 70, no. 2, p. 120-121.

Lempert, L. B. *Women's Health State from a Woman's Point of View: A Review of Literature.* : Hemisphere Publishing Company, 1980.

Miles, Agnes. *Women, Health and Medicine.*: Open University Press, 1991.

Miller, Connie and Leppa, Carol J. (eds.) *Women's Health Perspectives: An Annual Review.* USA: Oryx Press, 1988.

Mintz, Morton. *At Any Cost: Corporate Greed: Women and the Dalkon Shield.* New York: Pantheon Press, 1985.

Mitter, Swasti. *Common Fate, Common Bond: Women in the Global Economy.*: Pluto Press, 1991.

Morgan, Myfanwy et al. *Sociological Approaches to Health and Medicine.*: Croom Helm, Australia. 1985, Chap.1.

Nathanson, C.A. "Social Roles and Health Status Among Women: the Significance of Employment." *Social Science and Medicine.* : 1980 14 A (6), 463.

Navarro, V. *Medicine Under Capitalism.* New York: Neale Watson Academic Publication Inc.,1976.

Navarro, Vicente. *Imperialism, Health and Medicine.* :Baywood Publishing Company Inc., 1981.

———. "The Underdevelopment of Health or the Health of Underdevelopment." *Imperialism, Health and Medicine.* London: Pluto Press, 1982, p.15-36.

Petchesky Pollock, Rosalind. *Abortion and Women's Choice:The State, Sexuality and Reproductive Freedom.* New York: Longman, 1984.

Ratcliff Strother, Kathryn. "Health Technologies: Political and Ethical Considerations." *Healing Technology: Feminist Perspectives.* :University of Michigan Press, 1989, p. 173-194.

Smyke, Patricia. *Women and Health.* London: Zed Books Ltd., 1991.

Turshen, Meredith. *Women and Health in Africa.* USA: Africa World Press, 1991.

Whelehan, Patricia & Contributors. *Women and Health: Cross-Cultural Perspectives.* Massachusetts: Bergin & Garvey Publishers, Inc., 1988.

White, Kevin. "Trend Report, The Sociology of Health and Illness." *Current Sociology.* :Autumn 1991, Vol. 29, No. 2.

WHO Offset Publication. *Women, Health and Development.* Geneva: 1985, No.90.

Stellman, J.M., & Dawn, S. *Work is Dangerous to Your Health,* New York: Vintage Books, 1973.

Stellman, Mager Jeanne. "Women's Work, Women's Health." *Myths and Realities.* New York: Pantheon Books, 1977.

Yanoaskik, Kim & Norsigan, Judy. "Contraception, Control, and

Choice: International Perspectives." (ed.) Kathryn Strother Ratcliff *Healing Technology: Feminist Perspectives*.: 1989.

5. Health Issues (Caribbean Women)

Antrobus, Peggy. "Women, Health and Development." paper presented to the Distinguished Lecture Series, Trinidad and Tobago: PAHO/WHO, 1990. 9

Barroso, Carmen. *Women, Health and Development*. paper for PAHO Technical Discussion. Washington, D.C.:1988.

Hawkins, Irene. *The Changing Face of the Caribbean*. Barbados: Cedar Press Production, 1976.

Gish, Oscar. *Doctor Migration and World Health*. London: G.Bell & Sons, York House.

Hagley, Knox. "Nutrition and Mortality Trends in the Caribbean Region." *Cajanus*: 1987, Vol. 20.

LeFranc, E.R.M. *Health Status and Health Services Utilization in the English-Speaking Caribbean*. Kingston, Jamaica: ISER, 1990, Vol.11.

Massiah, J. "Work in the Lives of Caribbean Women." *Social and Economic Studies* : 1986, 35:177.

Musgrove, P. "The Economic Crisis and its Impact on Health and Health Care in Latin America and the Caribbean." *International Journal of Health Services*. 1987, Vol.17, No.3.

Reid, Una V. "Socio-economic Factors and the Impact on Women, Health and Development." paper presented in St. Vincent, Lucia, Barbados: PAHO/WHO, 23-27, 1990.

Sinha, Dinesh P. *Children of the Caribbean 1945-1984*: CFNI PAHO/WHO in collaboration with UNICEF, 1988.

Sunshine, Catherine A. *The Caribbean: Survival, Struggle and Sovereignty*.: An EPICA Publication, 1988.

Taylor, Le Roy. *Economic Adjustments and Health Care Financing in the Caribbean*. Jamaica: ISER, 1990.

World Bank Country Economic Report:1990.

World Development Report:1990, Vol. 1, No. 3.

Appendix 1

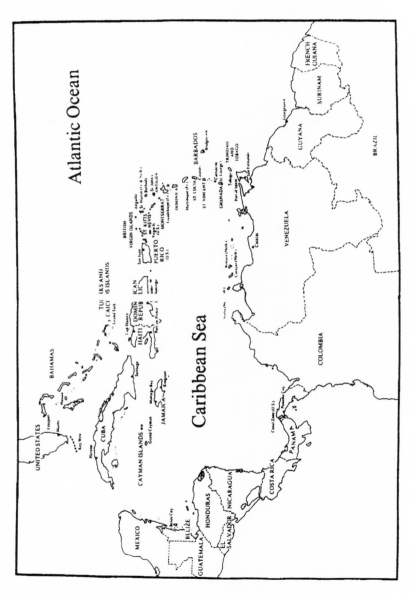

Map of the Caribbean

Appendix 2

Integrated Holistic Health System Components/Elements Model

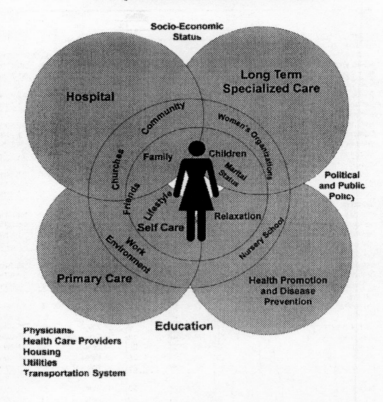

Appendix 3

**DETAILED DEMOGRAPHIC PROFILE OF THE
BARBADIAN AND GRENADIAN WOMEN INTERVIEWED**

	Barbadian		Grenadian		Total	
	No.	%	No.	%	No.	%
Women Interviewed	27	45.00%	33	55.00%	60	100.00%
Age Distribution						
30-39 years	11	40.74%	22	66.67%	33	55.00%
40-49 years	7	25.93%	6	18.18%	13	21.67%
50-55 years	9	33.33%	5	15.15%	14	23.33%
Race						
Black	26	96.30%	32	96.97%	58	96.67%
Indian	1	3.70%	1	3.03%	2	3.33%
Family Status						
Married	15	55.56%	5	15.15%	20	33.33%
Common Law	4	14.81%	1	3.03%	5	8.33%
Widowed	3	11.11%	1	3.03%	4	6.67%
Single	5	18.52%	26	78.79%	31	51.67%
Support Systems						
Had a person to confide in	22	81.48%	32	96.97%	54	90.00%
Confided in God	0	0.00%	1	3.03%	1	1.67%
No support	5	18.52%	0	0.00%	5	8.33%
Education						
Primary	26	96.30%	15	45.45%	41	68.33%
Secondary	2	7.41%	3	9.09%	5	8.33%
Polytechnic	2	7.41%	0	0.00%	2	3.33%
Continuing Education	0	0.00%	0	0.00%	0	0.00%
Employment Status						
Employed	23	85.19%	25	75.76%	48	80.00%
Self-employed	3	11.11%	1	3.03%	4	6.67%
Unemployed	1	3.70%	7	21.21%	8	13.33%
Housing						
Owned home/home & land	12	44.44%	24	72.73%	36	60.00%
Rented	23	85.19%	9	27.27%	32	53.33%
Telephone	27	100.00%	9	27.27%	36	60.00%
Electricity	27	100.00%	12	36.36%	39	65.00%
Piped water	26	96.30%	28	84.85%	54	90.00%
Indoor toilet	26	96.30%	28	84.85%	54	90.00%
Piped water & indoor toilet	26	96.30%	23	69.70%	49	81.67%
Religion						
Roman Catholic	0	0.00%	33	100.00%	33	55.00%
Christians	8	22.22%	0	0.00%	6	10.00%
Non - affiliation	21	77.78%	0	0.00%	21	35.00%

INDEX

Ability to Pay, 132, 189, 191

Abortion, 124

Abortion Law, 124

Adams, Sir Grantley, 109-110, 113

Adams, Tom, 113-114, 118, 120, 131, 135, 141

Adult Suffrage, 100-102, 145

Africa, 13, 19, 24, 33, 87-88

African States, 14, 24, 49

Agriculture, 23, 25, 56, 104, 154, 157, 187

Agro-industrial Enterprises, 157

AIDS, 241

Al-Naqeeb Kladoun Hassan, 29

Alavi, Hamza, 23, 48

Alma Ata Declaration, 76, 128, 139

Alleyne, Candia, 180

Alleyne, George A.O., 229

Ambursley Fitzroy & Dunkerley James, 141, 178-179

Amerindians, 90

Anarchist, 10

Animal and Human Health Programs, 138

Annual Reports, 79, 83

Ante-natal Care, 105, 194

Anti-colonial Struggles, 35, 63

Antigua, 39, 87, 117, 156

Antigua & Barbuda, 87, 117, 156

Antinatalist Policy, 66, 264

Antrobus, Peggy, 202

Apprentice, 94-95

Apprenticeship, 75, 90, 94-95, 107

Asians, 91

Armstrong, Pat & Armstrong, Hugh, 19

Australia, 33, 97

Authoritarian Rule, 37, 40

Authoritarian State, 28-29, 48-49, 148

Barbados, 2, 19, 58, 62, 71, 76-87, 89, 93, 95, 97, 99-100, 103, 105-106, 108-121, 123-125, 127-135, 137-143, 146, 156, 159, 163, 166, 183, 185-187, 189, 191, 193, 195, 197, 199-205, 207-211, 213-215, 217, 219, 221-223, 225, 227, 229-235, 238-242

Barbados Association of Medical Practitioners (BAMP), 83, 134-137

Barbados Community College, 138

Barbados Development Plan, 130, 141-142, 202, 234

Barbados Drug Service, 132

Barbados Labor Party (BLP), 81, 109-111, 230

Barbados Progressive League (BPL) Barbados Workers Union (BWU), 10

Barrett, Michele, 12, 16, 18-19

Barrow, Errol, 110-111, 141, 146

Beckles, Gloria, 88, 105

Beckles, Hilary, 80, 93, 106-107, 112, 140-142, 243

Belgium, 33

Belize, 87, 117, 156
Bishop, Maurice, 149, 153, 160, 164, 174
Bishop's Model, 114
Black Power Movement, 146
Bolles, Lynn, 82
Bourgeoisie, 7, 23, 25, 28, 30, 32, 34, 38, 41, 43-44
Brereton, Bridget, 54-55, 71
Bridgetown, 79, 223
British, 41, 49, 77, 94, 97, 100-103, 106-107, 113, 145, 147, 238
British Commonwealth, 94, 103
British Guiana, 100-101, 107
Brizan, George, 178
Bureau of Women's Affairs, 80, 85, 122, 142
Bureaucracy, 24, 41, 154, 183, 190, 213
Burnham, Forbes, 37
Burstyn, Varda, 13,18-19, 142
Bush, Barbara, 72

Callaghan, James, 113
Campbell, Bonnie, 26, 49, 56
Campbell, Horace, 28, 48
Canada, 91, 97, 136, 157, 199, 201
Canadian Imperial Bank of Commerce, 157
Cancer, 132, 188, 241
Capitalism, 3, 11-13, 22, 25-27, 29, 31, 36-37, 39, 42-43, 62, 66, 69, 237
Capitalist Society, 1, 6, 12, 16, 18, 21, 90
Capitalist State, 1, 3, 5-7, 9, 11-13, 15, 17-19, 21-22, 26, 31, 36-37, 237-238
Caribbean, 1-2, 4, 6, 8, 10-14, 16, 18-19, 21-22, 24, 26, 28, 30, 32, 34-40, 42-50, 53-73, 75-82, 84, 86-108, 110-118, 120, 122, 124, 126, 128, 130, 132, 134, 136-138, 140-142, 146, 148-150, 152-154, 156-158, 160, 162, 164, 166-168, 170,

172, 174, 176, 178-180, 184, 186, 188, 190, 192, 194-196, 198, 200, 202, 204, 206, 208, 210, 212, 214, 216, 218, 220, 222, 224, 226, 228, 230, 232, 234, 238, 240, 242
Caribbean Community and Common Market (CARICOM), 111, 167
Caribbean Contingency Joint Task Force, 113
Caribbean Development Bank (CDB) Caribbean Free Trade Association (CARIFTA), 111
Caribbean Labour Council (CLC), 110
CARICOM Partners, 156
Carriacou, 84, 165-167, 170, 175, 177, 225, 227
Carty, Linda, 19, 238
Cave Hill Campus of UWI, 111
Central Committee, 151, 161-162
Charles, Eugena, 39
Chauvinism, 34, 195
Chief Medical Officer of Health, 79-80, 87, 129, 140, 143, 190
Child Care Board, 120
Chile, 48, 148
China, 171, 239
Cholera, 95
Civil Rights, 30
Classism, 228, 233
Clement, Connie, 201
Coard, Bernard, 148, 152, 158
Coard, Phyllis, 161-162, 180
Codrington College, 120
Colonial Development and Welfare Act, 101
Colonial Development and Welfare Funds, 102
Coloured, 96
Columbus, 90, 107
Commandist State, 28, 48
Committee of Twenty-two, 146-147
Commonwealth, 73, 94, 103, 112, 234
Communal, 63
Communicable Diseases, 98, 102

Communism, 149
Community-based Primary Health Care, 171
Community Development, 80, 103, 111, 122, 142, 160, 170, 197
Community Health, 103, 162, 168, 172, 174, 177, 192, 195-197, 230, 239
Community Health Aides (CHA), 172
Community Health Nurses, 168, 174, 195, 239
Community Participation, 132, 168, 171, 197, 199, 229-230, 241
Connell, (Bob) R.W., 9, 10, 11, 18
Constitutions, 30, 40
Continuity of Care, 196, 225, 227, 229, 233
Costa Rica, 97
Cottingham, Jane, xix
Coups, 30
Crow, Ben, 22, 47, 49
Cuba, 35, 97, 149, 171, 174, 239
Cuban Medical Brigade, 167, 173
Curative, 126, 139, 163, 171, 216
Curative Care, 139, 163
Cypher, James, 25-26, 48

Dahlekrup, Drude, 17, 19
Dale, Roger, 33, 49
Dann, Graham, 129, 142-143
Davis, Angela, 19
De Riggs, Chris, 168, 170, 180
Diaspora, 82, 87-88
Disease, 91, 93, 187-189, 199, 241
Democracy, 32, 44, 46, 48, 50, 147-148, 178
Democratic Labour Party (DLP), 81, 110, 120, 230
Democratic Socialism, 42, 50
Depo Provera, 185
Depression, 34, 198
Despotic State, 7, 29
Development Plan, 104, 124, 130-131, 141-143, 174, 190, 201-202, 234

Diabetes, 132, 166, 210, 224, 241
Disempowerment, 92, 240
District Health Councils (DHC), 199
District Medical Officer, 166, 177
Domestic Labor, 57, 59, 69
Domestic Production, 10, 16, 69
Domestic Violence, 57, 198
Domicile Reform Act, 121
Domination, 5, 7, 9-10, 13, 16, 22-23, 27, 30, 33-35, 40-42, 50, 56-57, 59, 63-64, 97, 154
Dominica, 40, 78, 87, 117, 141, 156
Doyal, Lesley, xvii
Dumcasta Clause, 158

Elderly Phase, 133
Elite, 15, 24, 29, 50, 109, 112-113, 119, 125
Emancipate, 34
Emancipation, 14, 75, 90, 94-96, 98, 107
Emancipation Act, 96, 107
Emergency Powers Bill, 118
Emigration, 100, 157, 173
Emmanuel Patrick, 50
Empowerment, 137, 229, 242
Engles, Frederick, 12
Enslavement, 90
Essential Services and Port Authority Acts, 149
Ethiopia, 35
Ethno-cultural Groups, 92
Etter-Lewis, Gwendolyn, 82, 87
Europe, 33, 37, 136, 157
European Development Bank, 154
European Development Fund, 167
Exploitation, 12-13, 16, 22, 33-35, 41, 59, 62-64, 66, 70, 89, 93, 95, 158, 161
Extended Family, 92, 192

Family Care, 195, 198, 204, 206
Family Life Educators, 138
Family Planning Association, 185
Farrell, Trevor, 38, 39

Fascism, 34-35
Fatton, Robert, 14, 19
Fee-for-service, 126, 136, 191-192,
    233
Female-headed household, 104
Feminism, 11-12, 15-16, 18-19, 59,
    61, 87
Feminist, 1, 11-19, 47, 54-56, 59, 63,
    70, 73, 87, 190, 238
Fertility, 57, 66, 234
Feudalism, 28
Fields, Gairy S., 115-116, 141
Film Censorship Board, 120
Firearms Act, 149
Five Year Development Plan, 104, 124
Forde, Norma, 120-121, 123, 125,
    142
Forde-Smith, Honor, 238
France, 33, 35
Frank, Andre Gunder, 49
French, Joan, 238

Gairy, Eric Matthew, 145, 240
Gairyism, 168
Garvey, Marcus, 64-65
GDP, 115-117, 154, 157, 167, 169
Gender, 5, 9-14, 16-17, 19, 28, 36,
    44, 46-47, 53, 55, 57-62, 67,
    71-72, 86-87, 91, 96, 99, 104,
    124, 159, 176, 184, 187-189,
    198, 200, 220, 229, 232, 242
General Practitioner Service, 132-133
Germany, 34-35
Ghana, 45
Gillings, Scarlette L., 122-125, 142
Graham, Hilary, 202
Gramsci, Antonio, 617
Grass Roots, 170
Great Britain, 33, 35, 202
Green, Cecilia, 63-68, 72-73, 106
Grenada, 2, 39-40, 57-58, 62, 76-82,
    84-87, 89, 99, 103, 105-106,
    108, 114, 117, 141, 145-159,
    161, 163-181, 183, 185-187,
    189, 191, 193, 195, 197, 199-

201, 203, 205-211, 213-215,
    217, 219, 221, 223, 225, 227,
    229-235, 239-242
Grenada Bank of Commerce, 157
Grenada United Labour Party (GULP),
    145-149, 154, 168
Grenadian Socialism, 39
Grenadines, 87, 117, 156
Guadeloupe, 113
Guyana, 29, 35, 37, 39, 43, 50, 87,
    100, 102-103, 105, 108, 110,
    141, 151, 156, 234

Hagley, Knox, 266
Haniff, Yusif, 118, 141
Harley, Sharon, 82, 87-88
Hart, Richard, 110
Health Care System
    70, 81, 85, 101, 125, 128,
    131, 139, 163, 166, 170-172,
    175-176, 184, 186-187, 200,
    203, 213-214, 223, 230, 239
Health Centres, 101-102, 104, 126,
    133, 164-168, 170
Health Education, 78, 101, 103-104,
    106, 121, 138-139, 164, 167-
    168, 170, 174, 186, 200, 216,
    219-221, 229-231, 241-242
Health Education Division, 138
Health Education Officer, 138
Health Education Unit, 138
Health Educators, 105, 138, 174
Health For All by the Year 2000, 129,
    187
Health Policy, 2, 76-78, 81-83, 85, 87,
    89, 92, 130, 136, 142, 169-
    171, 183, 193, 199, 213, 235,
    240-241
Health Stations, 84, 164, 166-167,
    214, 218, 222
Health, Women and Development Plan
    Health Unit, 101
Hegemony, 3, 7, 11, 14, 151
Henry Forde, 120-121
High Blood Pressure, 210

Higman, B.W.,, 65
Hintzen, Percy, 43, 44, 50
Hookworm, 99, 102
House of Assembly, 119-120, 142
Human Resource Development, 174

Illiteracy, 100, 157
Illness, 91, 131, 199, 216, 229
Immunization, 104, 166
Imperial Act of Parliament, 94
Imperialism, 27-28, 30, 34, 38, 43,
          45, 48-49, 63
Imperialist, 27, 33-35, 41, 56, 119
Incomes and Prices Policy, 115-116
Indecency with Children Act, 121
Indentured, 56, 77, 97
Independence, 15, 17, 22-24, 27-28,
          34, 37-40, 42, 44, 46, 71, 75,
          90, 100, 102-103, 111-112,
          114, 147-148, 152
India, 44
Indo-Caribbean, 56
Industrialization, 30-31
Inequality, 13, 62-63, 92, 124, 141,
          176
Infant Mortality Rate, 79, 99
Infanticide, 90, 94
Instrumentalist Theory, 25
Inter-American Foundation (IAF), 80
Inter-Ministerial Group, 187
International Development Research
          Centre (IDRC), 80
International Economic Order, 155
Italy, 34
Ivory Coast, 36, 49

Jagan, Cheddie, 110
Jamaica, 39-40, 49-50, 71, 87, 95,
          99-100, 102-105, 107-108,
          110, 117, 128, 141, 156, 178,
          234
James, C.L.R., 267
Japan, 33-34
Jehovah Witness, 211
Jessop, Bob, 18

Joseph, Rita, 179-180, 234
Jules, Didacus, 79, 150-151, 153, 178-
          180

Kaiser Foundation International, 135
Keith and Keith, 42, 50, 234
Kellogg Foundation, 238

Labour Welfare Fund, 110
Latin America, 49, 58, 61, 72, 179
League of Nations, 33
Legislative Assembly, 119
Lesser Developed Countries (LDC), 78,
          114, 155
Lewis, Gordon K., 106, 108, 140
Liberal, 10, 12, 16-17, 78
Liberalism, 6, 16
Liberation Movements, 33
Life Expectancy, 79, 104-105, 136
Low-income, 241

MacKinnon, Catherine, 5, 12, 18-19
Macro-Political, 9
Magdoff, H., 49
Malaria, 102
Malnutrition, 93-94
Manifesto, 132, 136, 147
Manley, Michael, 39, 141
Mansour, Fawzy, 27, 48
Manufacturing, 114, 117, 154
Maroons, 96, 107
Marriage Act, 121
Marryshow House, Grenada School of
          Continuing Studies, UWI, 83
Marx, Karl, 12
Marxism, 12, 16, 19
Marxist, 6-7, 9-10, 12, 16-18, 58-59,
          110, 114, 149
Marxist-Leninist, 149
Masculinist, 65, 69, 125, 238
Massiah, Jocelyn, 107-108, 179, 201-
          202
Maternal and Child Health (MCH), 133
Maternal and Child Health Services,
          126, 133

Maternity Leave Law, 160
Medical Officer of Health (MOH), 173, 187, 188
Medical Termination of Pregnancy Act, 124, 142
Mental Health, 91, 94, 121, 125, 138, 216, 241
Merchant-planter Elite, 109
Metropolis, 13, 41
Michel-Rolph, Trouillot, 22, 47
Micro State, 78
Midwives, 105, 139, 166, 177
Migration, 38, 98
Miliband, Ralph, 3, 6
Minister of Tourism, 157
Minister of Tourism, Civil Aviation and Women's Affairs, 122
Ministry of Community Development and Culture, 80
Ministry of Employment, Labour Relations and Community Development, 80, 103, 111, 122, 142, 197
Ministry of Health, 83-84, 87, 104, 126, 129, 131, 140, 142-143, 163, 173, 185, 187-188, 192, 201, 234
Ministry of Housing, Land, Community and Culture, 122
Ministry of Information and Culture, 122
Ministry of Labour and Community Services Ministry of Transport, Works and Community Services, 122
Ministry of Women's Affairs, 80, 142, 160, 187
Mixed Economy Model, 155, 176
Mongoose Gang, 149
Monopoly, 25, 29, 45
Montserrat, 117
More Developed Countries (MDC), 78, 114
Morrissey, Marietta, 62, 72
Moyne Commission, 97, 101, 110

Moyne Report, 99, 107
Mozambique, 171
Multiparty Politics, 37
Munroe, Trevor, 40

National Commercial Bank (NCB), 157
National Commission on the Status of Women (NCSW), 120
National Democratic Congress (NDC), 81, 186, 224
National Drug Service, 239
National Executive Council, 120
National Health Legislation, 101, 121
National Health Service (NHS), 132-137, 239
National School Students' Council and Pioneers, 152
National Women's Organization (NWO), 84, 152, 159, 161, 213
National Youth Organization (NYO), 152
Nationalist, 37, 44, 65, 102
Nationalization, 27, 29, 32, 147
Nazi, 34
Neo-Colonialism, 31, 41, 44
Neo-Fascist, 30
Neo-Marxist, 10
Nevis, 78, 87, 98
New Jewel Movement (NJM), 146
New Zealand, 33, 97
Newspaper Act, 149
NHS Medical Practitioner, 132
NHS Model, 238-239
Nicaragua, 23, 48
Nigerian, 14, 19
Non-aligned Movement, 155
Non-Governmental Organization (NGO), 86, 120
North America, 37, 97, 185

O'Connor, James, 5, 18
October Socialist Revolution, 33
Offenses Against the Person Act, 124
Old Age Pension Plan, 118

Oligarchy, 28
Ollman, Bertell, 6, 18
Ontario Public Health Association
    (OPHA), 91-92
Oppression, 13, 16, 18, 34, 55, 59,
    68, 81, 91
Organization of American States (OAS),
    148
Organization of Petroleum Exporting
    Countries (OPEC), 155
Organization of Revolutionary Education
    and Liberation (OREL), 149
Organizing Committee (OC), 151
Ossification, 24
Out-Patient Department, 269

Pakistan, 28, 48
Panama, 97, 100
Pan-American Health Organization
    (PAHO), 81, 167
Parliamentary Representation, 40
Parish, 152, 158, 164, 172-173, 180,
    223
Parish Councils, 152, 158
Party Manifesto, 136, 147
Patois, 79
Patriarchal, 1, 10, 19, 57, 64, 69, 86
Patriarchal Societies, 57
Payne, Clement, 109
Peasantry, 32, 96
People's Law No. 29, 153
People's National Congress (PNC), 37,
    43, 151
People's National Movement (PNM),
    103
People's Progressive Party (PPP), 102
People's Revolutionary Army (PRA),
    150-151
People's Revolutionary Government
    (PRG), 84, 151, 161-166, 169,
    200, 213, 228, 230, 239
Peripheral Capitalism, 13, 22, 25-26,
    43, 69
Permanent Secretary, 171, 190
Petit Bourgeoisie, 28, 32, 38, 44

Petras, James, 30, 48
Pinochet, 148
Plantocracy, 77, 109
Pointe Saline, 154
Political Bureau (PB), 151
Polyclinics, 81, 83-84, 126-128, 132-
    134, 137-138, 166, 193, 214-
    215, 218-219, 222, 225-228,
    239
Poor Law System, 192
Porter, Rosemary Anne, 162
Post-Colonial, 1, 17, 21-24, 28, 30,
    32, 35-37, 44, 48, 57, 59, 71,
    78
Post-colonial Peripheral State, 1, 71
Post-colonial State, 1, 17, 21, 23-24,
    28, 32, 35-37, 48, 71, 78
Post-colonialism, 103
Post-natal Clinic, 166
Poulantaz, Nicos, 6
Poulantaz-Miliband Debate, 3, 6
Poverty, 34, 44-45, 56, 98, 103, 141,
    198, 211, 241
Power to the People, 137, 147
Pre-independence, 75, 90, 97
Prejudice, 11, 91
Pre-slavery, 90
Preventative, 105-106, 139, 163, 171,
    176, 216, 220
Primary Health Care (PHC), 76, 125-
    128, 131, 164, 166, 170
Princess Alice Hospital, 166
Princess Royal Hospital, 166
Productive Farmers' Union, 152
Project Design and Implementation
    Unit, 138
Proletariat, 43
Property Act, 121
Psycho-social, 168
Public Order Act, 149
Public Health, 84, 91, 98, 101, 104-
    106, 126, 137-138, 140, 163-
    164, 168, 172, 174, 177, 187,
    192-195, 200, 226
Public Health Educator, 138

Pulsipher, Lydia, 53, 71

Quality of Care, 220-221, 225, 227, 232-233, 239
Quasi-polygamous Unions, 64
Queen Elizabeth Hospital, 127-128, 134, 194

Racism, 32, 35, 56-58, 61, 63, 91-92, 102
Rastafarian, 113
Reagan Administration, 153
Reddock, Rhoda, 73, 235
Reductionism, 9
Reductionist, 16, 26, 59
Reid, Una, 270
Reforms, 37, 110, 122, 131
Repatriate, 34
Republicanism, 112
Retrenchment, 56
Revolutionary, 28, 78, 81, 98, 114, 149-152, 160-161, 168-169, 171, 174, 176
Robertson, C., 15
Rockefeller Foundation, 102
Rodney, Walter, 40, 50
Roman Catholic, 212
Roxborough, 26, 48
Royal Bank of Canada, 157
Royal Commission of Inquiry, 97
Russia, 33

Sanitation, 98, 102, 170
Seaga, Edward, 39
Second World War, 34, 41
Secondary Care, 106, 125-126, 133, 163, 166
Secondary Health Care (SHC), 125-126
Self Care, 199
Self-esteem, 91
Semi-proletarian, 23
Senior, Olive, 106-107
Service Accessibility, 214, 222, 233
Seventh Day Adventist (SDA), 211
Sexual Discrimination, 159

Sexual Harassment, 198
Sexually Transmitted Diseases (STD's), 241
Sexuality, 11, 16, 47, 57
Scott, J., 55
Sheridan, R.S, 93, 107
Simon, David, 48-49
Sinah, Dinesh P., 101, 117, 156, 195
Slave Trade, 91
Slavery, 46, 55, 58, 61-65, 75, 81, 90-96, 98, 106-107
Slaves, 63-64, 66, 72, 77, 89-94, 96-98, 106-107
Small Industry Credit Scheme, 154
Smallpox, 95
Smith, Adam, 63, 65
Smith, Dorothy, 18-19, 142
Special Benefit Service, 132
Social Services, 78, 103-104, 160, 170, 215
Socialism, 29, 35, 39, 42, 50, 110, 162
Socialist, 5, 10, 31, 33, 35, 39, 57-59, 106, 113-114, 146, 162, 171, 176, 239
Socialization, 8
Socio-economic, 2, 4, 15, 25, 39-40, 58, 61, 64, 70, 75, 85-86, 89, 95, 98, 105, 107, 114, 122, 125, 130, 145, 183, 204, 229, 242
Socio-political, 42
South Korea, 148
Soviet Union, 149
Spain, 90, 142
St. Christopher, 156
St. George's, 79, 135, 159, 167, 180, 185, 213, 223
St. George's General Hospital, 167
St. Joseph's Hospital, 126
St. Kitts, 87, 100
St. Lucia, 39, 78, 87, 100, 113, 117, 141
St. Vincent, 78, 87, 98, 100, 108, 113, 117, 141, 156

St. Vincent and the Grenadines, 87
Status of Children Reform Act, 121
Status of Women Council, 122
Status Quo, 96
Staudt, Kathleen, 19
Stephens Evelyn Hube & Stephens
John D, 41
Stock, and Anyinam,, 180
Stockdale, Sir Frank, 101, 148
Stone, Carl, 40, 50, 141, 143, 178
Stratification, 59-60, 62, 72
Stratification Theory, 59
Structural Adjustment Policies (SAPs),
210
Suicide, 90
Sunshine, Catherine A., 162, 211
Symke, Patricia, xvii

Tanzania, 146, 171
Taylor, LeRoy, 87, 141-142
Technocrats, 173
Tertiary Care, 106, 125-126, 129,
133, 163, 166, 193, 240
Tertiary Health Care, 125, 129, 163,
240
Testament Church of God, 212
Third World, 3, 13, 15, 19, 21-22, 24-
33, 35-37, 43-44, 47-49, 61-
62, 69-70, 149, 185
Thomas, Clive, 37, 40, 45, 103, 49-
50, 107-108, 141, 143, 180,
243
Tourism, 80, 114, 117, 124, 147,
154, 156-157, 238
Trade Unions, 81, 83, 108, 118, 153,
158
Traditional Healing, 92
Traditional Practitioners, 171
Transnational Corporations (TNC), 24
Transnationals, 27
Trinidad, 50, 71, 87, 99-100, 102-
105, 107-108, 114, 117, 141-
142, 156
Trinidad and Tobago, 71, 87, 103-104
True Blue Army, 150

Tuberculosis, 98, 102, 167
Tucker, J., 72

UN Resolution on the Discrimination of
Women, 160
Underdevelopment, 41, 48-49, 62, 89
Underemployment, 99
Unemployment, 34, 38, 44, 98-99,
101, 103, 114-119, 121-122,
139, 146, 155, 157, 209
Unemployment Benefit Scheme, 118-
119
UNESCO, 155
UNICEF, 79, 81, 87, 102
Union Island, 113
Union of South Africa, 33
United Nations (UN), 148
United Negro Improvement Association
(UNIA), 65
United States, 6, 35, 111, 157
University of the West Indies (UWI), 155
US Agency for International
Development (USAID), 167
US State Department, 86
User-friendly, 229
User Fees, 126
USSR, 35

Vargas, V., 58, 61, 72
Venezuela, 167

Walby, 59-60
Walker, Anne, 178, 180
Wallerstein, Immanuel, 49
Weinensee, Mary, 199, 202
West Indian, 65, 71-72, 91, 100, 180
West Indies, 48-50, 63-64, 71, 78, 80,
83-84, 90, 101, 105-107, 111,
114, 137, 140-141, 155
West Indies Labour Congress, 101
Westminister Model, 153
Westwood, Sally, 61, 72
White, Averille, 234
Williams, Eric, 107-108
Williams, Dessima, 180

Wiltshire-Brodber, Rosina, 71
World Health Organization (WHO), 167
Wolff, James, 50
Women's Desk, 159-160, 213
Working-class Women, 71, 82-83, 139,
        146, 183
World Bank, 154, 179
World War I, 33, 102
World War II, 35, 37, 41

Yaws, 102

6626488

3 1378 00662 6488